Look at Him

Look at Him

Anna Starobinets

Translated by
Katherine E. Young

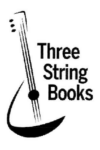

Three
String
Books

Bloomington, Indiana, 2020

Library of Congress Cataloging-in-Publication Data

Names: Starobinets, Anna, author. | Young, Katherine E. (Poet)
    translator.
Title: Look at him / Anna Starobinets ; translated by Katherine E. Young.
Other titles: Posmotri na nego. English
Description: Bloomington, Indiana : Three String Books, 2020.
Identifiers: LCCN 2020020363 | ISBN 9780893575038 (paperback)
Subjects: LCSH: Starobinets, Anna,--Health. |
    Pregnancy--Complications--Patients--Russia (Federation)--Biography. |
    Fetus--Abnormalities--Patients--Russia (Federation)--Biography. |
    Genetic disorders in pregnancy--Patients--Russia
    (Federation)--Biography. | Perinatal death--Psychological aspects. |
    Stillbirth--Psychological aspects.
Classification: LCC RG627.2.R8 S7313 2020 | DDC 618.20092 [B]--dc23
LC record available at https://lccn.loc.gov/2020020363

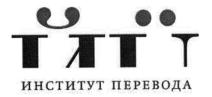

ИНСТИТУТ ПЕРЕВОДА

AD VERBUM

Published with the support of the Institute for Literary Translation (Russia)

Slavica Publishers   [Tel.] 1-812-856-4186
Indiana University   [Toll-free] 1-877-SLAVICA
1430 N. Willis Drive   [Fax] 1-812-856-4187
Bloomington, IN 47404-2146   [Email] slavica@indiana.edu
USA   [www] http://www.slavica.com/

Contents

Part 2. Others

Contents   vii

TRANSLATOR'S NOTE

The nomination of Anna Starobinets' *Look at Him* for the 2018 National Bestseller Award (the book was eventually named a finalist for the award) was greeted with controversy in Russia. In a strongly worded review ("as a human being, as a woman, I am physically sickened by this text"), Agalya Toporova complained that the book demonstrates "neither intelligence nor taste." Some attacked Starobinets for giving ammunition to antiabortion activists and religious zealots, for criticizing overworked and underpaid Russian medical practitioners, for envying women living through healthy pregnancies, and even for displaying her own privilege in seeking medical treatment abroad. Others charged that the author's description of her own suffering violates Russian social norms of stoicism; some derided the book for being maudlin or "anti-feminist." Literary critic Galina Yusefovich, on the other hand, called the book "a most important statement on a topic that no one has ever spoken aloud [in Russia]—necessary, traumatic, but also healing reading for any woman, and also for any man living with a woman and contemplating having children with her." Clearly, Starobinets had struck a nerve.

During the Soviet period, women living in the USSR commonly underwent multiple abortions over the course of their reproductive lives because most lacked access to other means of birth control. But in 2003, post-Soviet Russia—facing a falling birthrate, as well as the political resurgence of the Russian Orthodox Church—outlawed abortion after the twelfth week of pregnancy, except in cases of rape, imprisonment, death or disability of the husband, or loss of parental rights. Nevertheless, as detailed in this memoir, abortion continues to play a central role in women's reproductive life in Russia, not just as birth control up to the twelfth week of pregnancy but in response to the detection of birth defects much later in pregnancy.

Family planning, prenatal, and postnatal care services in Russia are offered, free of charge, to all women through the Russian Ministry of Health: the access point for this system of care is the local gynecological clinic (*zhenskaya konsultatsiya*) in the neighborhood where a woman is registered as living. However, there is widespread dissatisfaction with the quality of services provided under this system. Like Anna Starobinets, many women who can afford it seek private care, which they pay for out of their own pockets. Private, paid care, which is available primarily in Russia's cities, may be offered by clinics that serve only private clients, or by public institutions that offer various paid options in addition to the free services mandated by the Ministry of Health. The continuing evolution of this system is evident even in this memoir, which notes in passing that the services offered by Moscow's Kulakov Research Center changed as Starobinets was writing her book.

Maternal and fetal health care practices change quickly, too, and what was standard medical practice in 2012, when the events described in this memoir took place, may no longer be the norm. No attempt has been made in this translation to note or correct medical or scientific errors in the original text. For example, in Chapter 12, Starobinets states categorically that abortions by caesarian section are not possible in the second trimester, a fact that may have been true in 2012, but is apparently no longer the case. Similarly, the professional titles recorded by Starobinets for the various Russian and German medical personnel she contacted date to the period when she contacted them; many have attained higher professional rank since this book was written.

Aside from its artistic, social, and cultural importance in Russia, *Look at Him* addresses issues that are central to the discussion of abortion anywhere in the world, including in the United States. In her unflinching portrayal of the anguish faced by the parents of a child whose medical condition means that he won't live past birth—a child who will, in fact, die in excruciating pain—Starobinets cuts to the heart of what medicine can and cannot do. In chronicling her own decision about such a pregnancy, Starobinets bravely divulges her doubts about that decision, as well as her horror at its consequences.

Heartfelt thanks are due to my friend and colleague Lisa C. Hayden, whose review of the Russian original of *Look at Him* on her blog about Russian literature, *Lizok's Bookshelf*, introduced me to this magnificent and heartbreaking book. Lisa was also kind enough to introduce me to the agents for Starobinets—Banke, Goumen & Smirnova Literary Agency—when we all found ourselves in Moscow in 2018. Poet and translator Bernadette Geyer offered crucial insight on German phrases in the original text, as well as information about Charité-Universitäts-medizin and about Berlin in general. Kathryn Dreger, MD, generously checked the manuscript's medical content, consulting with her professional colleagues when necessary; her advice has been invaluable. My indefatigable friend and colleague Liza Prudovskaya checked the English text against the Russian original, sometimes multiple times, offering valuable insights and suggestions along the way. Any remaining errors are mine alone.

Katherine E. Young
December 2019

FOREWORD

It's one thing to dream up scary stories and another thing entirely to become the main character of a horror tale yourself. For a long time, I doubted whether it was worth writing this book. It's really too personal. Too real-life. Not literature.

But all I know how to do is write. I have no other means to change the world. This book isn't just about my personal loss. This book is about how inhumane the system is into which a woman falls when she needs to terminate a pregnancy for medical reasons in my country. This book is about humanity and inhumanity in general.

What's lost can't be returned. You can't turn those who've lost their human form back into people. But you can correct the system, and I hope for that. That's why I name real names and institutions. That's why I write the truth.

It's possible that my hopes won't come to pass. That those who make decisions and spin the wheels in this system won't ever open my book. That some of those whose names I've named will experience nothing but anger. So be it.

But if this book helps someone who's grieving, that means it won't have been written in vain.

And it means that there was some kind of reason for what happened to us.

ACKNOWLEDGEMENTS

To my husband Sasha, who shared all this with me.
To my daughter Sasha, who became my consolation.
To Natashka, who led me through hell.
To my parents, who helped us escape.
To the doctors at the Charité clinic, who showed us humanity.
To all the friends who supported me.
To my unnamed son, who was with me for such a short time.
And to my second son Lev, who stayed with me.

PART 1

Us

CHAPTER 1
BIRTH DEFECT

"Well, is it a girl or a boy?" I ask the ultrasound specialist.

He's already been able to show me the brain, "The baby has a very good brain." And heart—"Everything's well developed there." He's already said the measurements correspond to sixteen weeks of development. He's already asked me the absurd question to which I've become accustomed over sixteen weeks, "Who have you got at home?" and I've already answered that I have an eight-year-old girl at home. So, this time I'd like a boy. And now I'm asking if it's a boy or girl, but for some reason he's pursing his lips tightly. As if he's got a giant, sour berry in his mouth and is deciding whether or not to spit it out. He silently guides the probe around my stomach and looks silently at the monitor. He's silent a little too long, and then he says, "It's a boy."

But something's wrong with his voice. With the tone. Again, he purses his lips. I suddenly remember the beginning of my own science fiction book, *The Living*: "The probe cheeped, and the doctor considered what he was seeing. I asked, 'Is something wrong?' He was silent. 'Is something wrong with the baby?'"

And now, it's November of 2012, and I myself am in the office of a doctor who is silent, and the ultrasound cheeps, and I ask, "Is something wrong with the baby?"

He resolves, finally, to get rid of his sour berry. "Does anyone in your family have kidney disease?"

"No...."

"I don't like the structure of the kidneys in this fetus. It's a hyperechogenic structure."

For a few seconds, I even feel relief. Kidneys, no big deal. Kidneys—well, that's important, of course, but it's not the heart, not the lungs, not the brain, he has a good heart and brain, but we can somehow treat the kidneys, especially as there's no hereditary kidney disease in the family. That's probably a good indicator for the prognosis...

"And they take up the greater part of the fetal abdominal cavity," he adds. "They're five times larger than they should be."

It's possible to not know what a hyperechogenic structure is, but it's absolutely clear that kidneys shouldn't take up the whole stomach. So, naturally, I understand that this is bad. Very bad.

"It's possible that the fetus has polycystic kidney disease," he says. "Wipe yourself off and get dressed."

It seems that at that moment, for the first time, I split in two. With shaking hands, one of me wipes the gel off my stomach. But the other me attentively and calmly watches the first, and the doctor as well, and she's generally quite observant. For example, she notices that he no longer calls my baby a baby. Just a "fetus."

"You need an ultrasound by an expert"—he writes the name of a clinic and a doctor's last name on a piece of paper—"preferably this doctor, he's a specialist in fetal birth defects."

I ask, "Is it very serious?"

He answers, but it's the answer to a different question. "I'm just an ultrasound doctor. I'm not an expert and not the Lord God, and I make mistakes. Go see an expert."

It seems to me that he also wants to add "And pray," but he doesn't say anything more.

It's said the first stage of grief is denial. Having learned terrible news, it's as if you can't immediately take it in. You maintain that it's just a mistake, or that they're knowingly lying to you, that the ultrasound doctor is a charlatan, that he's sending you to his friend for another ultrasound in order to take your money... Yes, I've seen that kind of thing in online chat rooms dedicated to the pathology of pregnancy, and even my mother, having learned the results of the ultrasound, passes through this stage very quickly, right before my eyes. It's a normal defense mechanism—but for some reason, it doesn't work for me. Even before I went online to read about polycystic kidney disease, even before the diagnosis was announced, in that moment when he looked at the monitor and was silent, I understood that things were very bad. Really bad.

I pay for the ultrasound and go out into the wet November darkness. I walk along the street, then I grasp that I'd come in a car, but I can't remember where I left it. For twenty minutes, I drag myself around the obstetrics and gynecology clinic on Bolshaya Pirogovka Street, forgetting what, exactly, I'm looking for. It's hard to walk. As if I'm moving inside a thick, black cloud. Eventually, I stumble upon my car, climb in, and go online on my phone. I type in "fetal polycystic kidney disease" and open up more and more links, and I understand that polycystic kidney disease occurs in two types, dominant (adult) and recessive (infantile). That dominant polycystic kidney disease is exactly the kind that runs in families, and that people generally live with it. But recessive is what we're talking about in my case. If it is my case. In the photographs, there are deformed infants with flattened faces and giant, inflated stomachs. Dead infants. They don't survive with infantile polycystic kidney disease.

... The thick, black cloud surrounding me suddenly begins to crawl into my mouth and my throat. I'm suffocating. There's absolutely nothing for me to breathe. The other me, the one who's cold and calm, notices then that I'm not simply sitting in the car and staring at the telephone screen gasping for breath, but am at the same time driving along Tenth Anniversary of October Street, and everyone's honking at me because I'm crawling into oncoming traffic.

By some miracle, I manage to drive home, all the same. I can't breathe, and when my daughter Sasha, we call her Little Badger, comes happily running with the question "Is it a boy or girl?" and my husband, also Sasha, comes out of the kitchen with wet hands and inquires offhandedly, "Is everything okay?" I can't speak and only gasp and gasp for air, but there is no air: my black cloud doesn't let it into my lungs.

"What's wrong with the baby?" Big Sasha grabs me by the shoulders. "What's wrong with our baby?"

Little Badger looks at us in fright and prepares to cry. The observant, calm me also looks at us, and reproachfully. She doesn't like the fact that we're scaring our daughter. She doesn't like the fact that I can't pull myself together. But it amuses her that we all seem to be playing a scene from a soap opera.

"I can't breathe," I sob, exactly as if I were fulfilling the conventions of the genre.

My husband brings me a small glass of whisky and says, "Drink it down."

Looking at my stomach, which hasn't been showing long at all, he adds, "Nothing bad will happen to the baby from such a tiny amount. Drink."

I swallow the contents of the glass, and I really do relax. I breathe, I look at Little Badger and Big Badger. Just this morning, we were discussing what the new baby's nickname would be. Sasha was afraid the baby would usurp her position of Little Badger, but I said we'd call the baby Littlest Badger, and no one would be offended... And now I say to them both, say to my badgers, "It's a boy. But he won't live. Probably."

For the rest of the night, my husband and I sit at the computer reading about polycystic kidney disease. From time to time I weep, but my husband tells me that nothing's definite yet, that we need to first wait for the ultrasound with the expert, that I'm panicking too soon. And Little Badger makes me a card with a drawing of a flower: "Mama, everything will be fine" is written on it, in the clumsy handwriting for which they scold her in school. And she also drags all her toys to me, one after the other, and says they'll be my talismans, that they'll protect me.

That same night, for the first time in sixteen weeks, the baby begins to stir inside me. They're soft, sliding movements—as if he's stroking me. As if we've all gathered together, the whole Badger family, except Big Badger and Little Badger are on the outside, and Littlest Badger is inside me. As if everything will be fine. Like in the movies.

Chapter 2
These Don't Survive

In the morning, Little Badger wakes up with a sore throat, so Big Badger stays with her. And I go alone to the V. I. Kulakov Research Center for Obstetrics, Gynecology, and Perinatology on Oparin Street. Last night, I managed to google Dr. Voyevodin— the one whose name is written on my paper—and Google made clear to me that he really is one of the best experts in the country. The reception desk tells me on the phone that Voyevodin won't take me, that he's booked for the next three weeks. But they have other specialists who are experts. It's hard to get an appointment with them on such short notice, too, but one can only try, so I should come.

I take a couple of talismans with me—a stuffed dog and a stuffed meerkat—and I go. I can't wait three weeks. At the Kulakov Center, there's an unbelievable number of women and a handful of men accompanying them. They sit in the waiting room and wait their turn. Almost all the women have gigantic stomachs. At a minimum, half of them are "preggy-weggies." While I'm looking for the reception desk, one preggy-weggy next to me tells another in a capricious voice, "I don't take hormones, just teensy-weensy vitamins. The most important thing is that itsy-baby-kins is comfortable in my belly-welly." Preggy-weggies (they call themselves that in women's chat groups) differ from women who are simply pregnant in their heightened sentimentality, their inclination to communicate in baby talk, and sometimes also in wearing pink jumpsuits for future mothers. In their stomachs sit itsy-bitsy babies and belly-dwellers. And they're quite comfortable there... But mine, no. Mine is probably uncomfortable. Because it's probably hard to be comfortable if your kidneys are five times larger than normal. And I'm uncomfortable. This waiting room looks like the waiting room at a train station. These women have the kind of face that it seems as if a toy train is going to come for them right here and carry them into a wonderful future. To baby formula, to pink and blue ribbons, to onesies and disposable diapers. And to little ones who have normal kidneys.

And I'm not getting on that train.

Is this envy? I'm not going to lie. It's envy.

I stand in line at the reception desk and say that I need an ultrasound by an expert.

"Are you pregnant?" The lady behind the desk is surprised. "How far along are you?"

I'm four months pregnant, but my stomach is barely showing. As if I weren't pregnant at all. It's even, somehow, disappointing.

"Sixteen weeks," I tell her. "Fetal polycystic kidney disease. Please."

The lady becomes more sympathetic and goes to see if anyone among the super-duper experts can take me today without an appointment.

A preggy-weggy in a pink track suit retreats a step from me, as if she's afraid she'll be infected by misfortune. The whole line stares gloomily, not exactly at me, but off to the side.

The lady comes back to the desk.

"Professor Demidov has agreed to see you. He's a luminary in the field. Will you take it? The ultrasound will cost three thousand rubles."

I take it. What's three thousand rubles? I'm prepared to pay even more. Yesterday's non-expert ultrasound on Pirogovka Street cost that much. I sit in the waiting room and enter "Demidov fetal ultrasound" in my smartphone. Wikipedia tells me that Vladimir Nikolayevich Demidov is "a Soviet and Russian doctor of obstetrics and gynecology and a perinatologist. A doctor of medical science. A professor. One of the founders of ultrasound and perinatal diagnostics in the USSR." In other words, truly a luminary.

I experience a rush of gratitude for the elderly professor who so easily, without any fuss, out of pure sympathy will see me on this very day, just like that. That's what being a doctor means, doctor with a capital "D." Old school, from the Soviet era. My number (the numbers are lit up on a display) is still a long way off, so I go looking for the toilet.

There's one bathroom on the floor—that is, a single toilet. If you're a man, or by chance a woman who's never been pregnant, perhaps you don't know that for pregnant women, the urge to urinate occurs quite often, and it's quite strong, first of all, for hormonal reasons and, second of all, because the growing uterus presses on the bladder. For that reason, standing in a line of fifteen people for the single toilet is quite agonizing. I write this not because I fail to understand why there's only one toilet (although I don't understand that), but because I want to be clear about the state I find myself in when my turn for the toilet finally arrives. I'm just about to grasp the door handle when my path is blocked by a cleaning lady with a bucket and mop. She literally blocks me—she stands in the doorway and doesn't let me enter. She looks down at my feet, at my winter boots, and on her face is hatred:

"Why aren't you wearing shoe covers?!"

Why am I not wearing shoe covers? I don't know. I hadn't thought about disposable shoe covers. I hadn't seen where to buy them.

I didn't know. I'm sorry.

"You didn't know. Go to the first floor and put on some shoe covers! You can't go into the toilet without shoe covers."

I understand that I won't make it to the first floor. That if now, this very second, I don't find myself in the blessed toilet, I will simply pee all over myself.

"I really need to use the toilet," I say to the cleaning lady. "Then I'll go immediately and get shoe covers."

"I won't let you without shoe covers," she answers.

Then I turn into an animal. I understand that I hate her. She hates me, and I hate her, we're two aggressive females, I'm no longer a medical patient, and she's not an employee: the loss of our common humanity takes place in an instant. She's the elder female, I'm the younger one. I'm obviously stronger than she is. For that reason, I simply push her out of the door of the toilet with both hands, rush inside, lock the door behind me and answer, as they say, the call of nature.

"You bitch, damn you..." The voice of the cleaning lady reaches me through the door.

Then I do indeed go down to the first floor and buy shoe covers. And I wait for my turn. My husband phones and says he's spoken with Professor Voyevodin's personal assistant and that she said I could go upstairs to his office and perhaps he'd see me. But I've already paid for an ultrasound with Demidov. And soon my number will light up. So, I stay and wait. Professor Demidov sees me after an hour.

He moves the probe around my stomach and mutters:

"So, the kidneys... Yes... That certainly looks like polycystic kidney disease... Or perhaps bilateral multicystic dysplastic kidney... So, the sex... It's a boy... A cephalic presentation... I want to examine the brain transvaginally...Undress to the waist..."

I undress. Demidov quietly converses about something with his assistant, I hear an indistinct muttering: "Of course... Who wouldn't be interested..."; then she leaves the room.

The professor inserts the transvaginal probe in my vagina.

After a minute, about fifteen people in white coats enter the room, escorted by the assistant—medical students and young doctors.

They line up along the walls and watch in silence. And I'm lying there, naked. With a transvaginal probe in my private parts. Once again, I split in two. The me who's on the edge of hysterics screws up her eyes so as not to see them and, it seems, weeps. The other me, observant and calm, reflects on how funny it is that the whole scene, both in feeling and setting, looks like a fragment of a nightmare. There's a common type of nightmare, for example, when you go up to the blackboard not wearing any underwear.

Then he pulls out the probe and moves the transducer around my stomach to demonstrate to the students what they'd missed.

"Look, such a typical picture," says Professor Demidov. "There are the cysts... See? There they are, many cysts... The size of the kidneys is five times larger than normal... The bladder is underdeveloped... Look, how interesting... For now, a normal amount of amniotic fluid... But soon there will be too little... With these kinds of defects, children don't survive..."

They don't survive. Don't survive. Don't survive.

Professor Demidov isn't addressing me, he's addressing the students. He doesn't notice me anymore. I don't exist anymore.

For a short while, the calm me takes over my body entirely. I lie without underwear, tears roll down my cheeks, these children don't survive, but all that is happening to someone else. And I'm reflecting on things.

I think that, purely for educational reasons, showing "a typical picture" to students and beginning doctors is important. That it's absolutely necessary for the education of qualified medical personnel. So they can distinguish one pathology from another. One cyst from another. And I understand that it's even better to show how a pathology looks using a live example. My example. But here's the really strange thing. If I'm now honestly serving medicine as a whole and the V. I. Kulakov Research Center for Obstetrics, Gynecology, and Perinatology in particular, why the hell did I pay three thousand rubles for this examination? And as I'd already paid, then why didn't the luminary of science simply ask me whether I objected to having a crowd of strangers observe me now? By the way, I'd most probably have agreed. For the same reason I'm writing this book—so that there might be just the tiniest practical benefit from what happened.

The most remarkable thing is that when I describe this scene the next day to my friend S, a pediatrician, he'll be sincerely surprised at my indignation. He'll say, "That's common practice. Students need to learn." And only when I remind him about the three thousand rubles and about ethics will he appear to agree with me—but, somehow, without full conviction.

And, by the way, about "common practice." Is it common that the professor, informing me about the fact that my baby won't survive, doesn't express any regret or sympathy? "I'm very sorry, but these children don't survive." That would have sounded better. Of course, the professor isn't sorry. The professor has a *déformation professionnelle*, and he saw me, probably, because my case could be used for pedagogical ends, but these are all questions having to do solely with the professor and his mental makeup. Here's what has to do with "common practice": the formal expression of sympathy in such situations is a norm of human relations. It's an international standard. A basic. In a few more days, I'll discover that we generally lack that kind of standard here in Russia. Sometimes, I come across people who consider it necessary to say, "I'm so sorry" or "I sympathize." But that's the exception. No generally accepted rituals for expressing compassion exist.

Maybe you think this isn't important. That it doesn't make anything easier. Believe me. It's important. And easier. Just a very little bit, but easier. Imagine you don't have any skin, that even the wind hurts you, that you hurt yourself. Now, imagine that someone touches you. Would you prefer that hand to be wearing a canvas work glove? Or would you prefer that the person who touches you first take off the glove, wash that hand with soap, and smooth it with cream?

"Get dressed," the professor says, his expression slightly perplexed. "Why are you sitting there? Wipe yourself off and get dressed."

I discover that I really am sitting vacantly on the table—without any underwear, with gel smeared across my stomach—and looking fixedly at one spot.

I wipe myself off and get dressed. The students silently observe me. In the absolute silence of the grave.

I break that silence:

"He won't live at all?"

"Well, maybe not 'at all,'" answers the professor. "Maybe he'll live a short while. Two or three days. Or even a month. It's up to you. Terminate the pregnancy or carry it to term."

"Where do I go now?"

"Go to your local gynecological clinic."

"But what about here?..."

"We don't deal with those things here."

This is the first time (but far from the last) that I hear the formulation "those things," but now, I'm too overwhelmed to prick up my ears.

"Thank you," I say to the professor.

It seems to me that some kind of human feeling flashes across his face, but he immediately banishes it deep.

"Go to the gynecological clinic," he repeats again, for some reason.

I leave the room and come face to face with that same cleaning lady. She silently casts a glance at me, and an entirely sincere, somehow even childlike expression of malicious pleasure spreads over her face. I don't know how I look. Very bad, I have to think.

What I do next—it's probably pure denial. Which finally comes over me. I don't go downstairs to the coat check room. I climb up to the floor where the expert Voyevodin sees patients. I don't fully make sense of my actions, but I want, I simply have to have, another ultrasound by an expert. And precisely by that doctor whose name is written on the paper. Because he's the absolute best. And he takes a modern approach. Not some moss-covered Soviet style. It's possible he'll say something different. I don't hope that he'll say everything's okay. But I hope he'll give me just some kind of chance. If only a low percentage. That my baby will be born and might live. We'll treat him. We'll do everything. A kidney donor, dialysis, everything we can...

I stand in line for Professor Voyevodin. It's already near evening, I wait while he sees the last patient on the list, and then I go in.

Voyevodin is typing on his computer keyboard.

"I'm busy," he says. "I didn't call you."

"When can I come?"

He turns his face to me, dissatisfied and self-satisfied at the same time.

"I'm a very busy man. What is it that you need?"

I begin to explain confusedly that my husband had phoned the assistant and that the doctor who'd done my ultrasound on Pirogovka Street had recommended I come to him and only him, and that the assistant had told me to come...

"Oh, that's you," he becomes slightly mollified, but then and there grows gloomy anew. "That was two hours ago. Why did you wait till now?"

I begin to cry. I say I'd already gotten an appointment with Demidov, that my turn in line had come, and that...

"So, you already had an ultrasound with Demidov?" Voyevodin bellows.

"Yes."

"Then what do you want from me?" Now he's really yelling. "They told you to come to me, you went to Demidov, you made your choice, what do you want now? Get out of here!"

"I want to you do an ultrasound."

"But you went to Demidov!"

"I'm sorry."

I feel like an earthworm who's been cut in two with a piece of glass. In two halves. One half wriggles around, demeans herself, and releases floods of tears and snot because she wants an ultrasound. The other half almost doesn't move. She despises the first half. And she whispers to her: "Don't you see that this man is a bastard?"

"What diagnosis did he give you?" asks Voyevodin.

"Bilateral multicystic dysplastic kidney."

"Length of pregnancy?"

"Sixteen weeks."

"My ultrasound costs a lot," he calms down slightly. "Six thousand rubles."

"Fine," I answer. "I have that."

"Then come back in two weeks. I like to look at the kidneys at eighteen weeks. I won't look now. Don't do anything for these two weeks. No invasive procedures. No abortion. Wait."

Of course, I don't go back to him. But later, I clarify that it wasn't simply out of caprice that he proposed coming back in two weeks. But because it really is better to examine the condition of the genitourinary system at eighteen weeks. If only because at that time, the fetal kidneys fully take on the function of filling the uterus with fluid (the embryo swallows the amniotic fluid and excretes it back in urine, it's a closed ecosystem), and if there's fluid, it means that kidney function has been at least partially preserved; if there's no fluid, it means that the kidneys don't work at all. Which is to say that, from the medical point of view, the expert Voyevodin was correct.

This doesn't cancel out the ugliness—from the human point of view—of what took place. However, the moral qualities of the expert are a problem that concerns just him and his family. But the lack of the requisite norms of behavior in a medical establishment—that's also a problem that concerns the system.

And once more about rituals. In sufficiently developed societies, there are thought-out, established formulas and even established intonations for such situations as mine and for many others—formulas that don't necessarily need to come from the heart, but that it's necessary to use in order to observe ethical practice. Most likely, a weeping lady who turns up in an expert's office at the end of the workday without an appointment, having beforehand done an ultrasound at a competitor's office, will evoke no less irritation in an expert in a developed society than in a less developed one. But in the developed society, the expert will respond with an established formula: that he trusts the opinion of a colleague, however, he's prepared, if desired, to give a *second opinion*, but today, alas, he's not seeing any more patients, call at such and such a time, come back at such and such a date. Here in Russia, these established formulas are lacking, and "improvised" formulas are produced from scratch in each concrete instance by each concrete individual. And they very much depend on whether the individual has been in a traffic jam, whether he has a headache, and whether he fought with his wife that morning.

Again, even in fully developed societies, an ultrasound expert, if his head really hurts, is fully capable of blowing a gasket for a little while, forgetting all formulas, and simply shouting at a woman at the top of his lungs. However, after such an event, the ultrasound expert most probably will be fired from the medical institution. Moreover, there will be a scandal. And a stain on his reputation. With regard to the expert Voyevodin, as far as I know, he's quite successful. His ultrasound costs a lot, and he's a very busy man.

... The two halves of my earthworm somehow manage to hold crookedly together, and for a long time I crawl around the V. I. Kulakov Research Center for Obstetrics, Gynecology, and Perinatology and can't find the coat check area. And then I can't find my claim check. And then I can't find the way out.

I want someone to take me by the hand and lead me out of there. But there isn't anyone.

Don't ever go to such places alone. Take your husband, or a friend, or the husband of a friend, your mother, uncle, sister, hell, the neighbor across the landing. Take anyone who'll help you find the way out. Not the ultimate way out, just the way out of the building.

CHAPTER 3
JUST A FETUS

Little Badger is an optimist. She believes that a miracle will happen for us and Littlest Badger will be born. For her, this is probably the stage of denial. But it's important to her that I believe as well, as if my faith could fix things. She follows me around like a shadow: "But don't you believe just a teeny bit? Don't miracles happen? Don't you believe even a smidge? Even one percent? Even a whisker?"

I don't know how best to answer her, so I say what I'm thinking. I don't believe. Not one percent, not a smidge, not a whisker. My stage of denial has already passed. Probably, it's cruel, but I don't want to give Little Badger hope. The more hope there is now, the worse it will be later.

They say the second stage of grief is anger.

It's not that I'm angry—but I want to know whose fault it is.

The main person, the one whose fault all of it is, is me. I run through these sixteen weeks in my head and find many sins. I didn't rejoice to the necessary degree at the conceiving of new life in me. The preggy-weggies write in online chat rooms: "When I saw those two cherished lines, my joy knew no bounds." That's their mantra. Their incantation. It's like the beginning of a prayer. As if there's a special deity who monitors their chat room and who must be appeased. And I didn't appease the deity. I did things wrong, in general. There were limits to my joy. When I saw the two lines on the test, I felt scared. It's true that at my first pregnancy, which resulted in Little Badger, I also felt scared, but that's not important. This time, I felt even more scared. Furthermore, I drank wine the night he was conceived. I smoked. I didn't eat regularly. I didn't go swimming. Worked too much. Wrote a new book. Wrote a screenplay. Wrote articles. And now I also need to write. Up until this nightmare began—that is, until three days ago—I was working on a long article, moreover, on deadline. But now I can't write anything. I send the editor-in-chief an email about birth defects and about the fact that I can't do anything right now. The response arrives: "Of course. We'll postpone it."

That article is about children the social service authorities want to remove from their family. Because their home is dirty, there are cockroaches, dogs, cats, rats, and fleas. Because the place stinks. Because their mama takes in every stray animal she sees. Because at some point, the social service authorities also took their mama from her own mama, and she grew up in an orphanage and has no understanding of what a normal home is. I wanted to stand up for them, to write that families can't be separated, that the vicious cycle of being an orphan must be broken. That these children are attached to one another and their mother, no matter what. And that they can't be taken away, that a social worker must work with them. That although they stink, they're happy. In an orphanage, they'll be clean and unhappy. I spoke with volunteers and psychologists. I visited them. In their stinking, vagrant hovel.

It's their fault. They infected me. I was there during the first trimester, at exactly the stage when the organs form. It's her fault, their criminal, dimwitted mother. She has four children and doesn't bother about any of them. How can she live in a dump but give birth to healthy children? How can her sons live and mine not survive?

Because I didn't have to visit them in their unsanitary state. It's my fault.

But then again, no. Polycystic kidney disease is a genetic illness, it's impossible to be infected with it. So, it's my fault, not because I visited that hovel, but for a different reason.

I know why. I committed a sin. The most important sin.

I once said I didn't want him. Didn't want a second child. I said that maliciously during a fight with Big Badger. Words have power. It was sometime during the eighth week. Probably at exactly the stage when the kidneys were forming.

Big Badger. It's his fault. His fault that I said that. And besides, he said the wrong words. He said it was a bad time. That we had too much work right now.

"You didn't want him!" I attack Big Badger. "You said he'd mess everything up! Well, are you happy now?"

Big Badger says:

"No, I'm not happy. In fact, I wanted him, too."

And he adds, helplessly:

"I wanted to play soccer with him."

I'm ashamed, but I want to keep picking at this some more:

"And now there won't be any baby. No baby."

And then he tries to persuade me that it's not a baby but a fetus. A fetus can't exist outside my body. A fetus doesn't yet live in the full meaning of the word... He argues. He insists. He wants to comfort me, but I fall into despair. My baby is alive, he kicks, he stirs around. I shout: "Don't you dare call him a fetus! He's a person!"

"Fine, but can I call him an embryo?"

"Embryo" sounds better. We conduct a teleological argument about the soul of an embryo. My husband, who was baptized in the Russian Orthodox Church, insists that an embryo probably doesn't have a soul. I, who was never baptized, insist that he has a soul. And that I feel that soul. An additional, pure soul inside of me.

"Fine," says Big Badger. "It's clearer to you."

He gives in simply to soothe me. He continually gives in to me and soothes me. He cooks, he goes to the store, he washes dishes, he prepares Little Badger's inhaler and gargle for her throat. He works, he begs me to eat, he hugs me and strokes my head and says: "I'm here." He talks on the phone with my parents and his parents. I lie around and weep but, like the wolf in the old video game, he tries to catch all the eggs in all the baskets. He's here. However, that little boy with enormous kidneys isn't inside him but inside me. It will fall to me to kill him very, very soon. Or else it will fall to me to carry him to term. And to watch as he dies.

CHAPTER 4
WE DON'T DEAL WITH THOSE THINGS

Mariya[1] The 22-week ultrasound showed that the baby had a congenital defect—Arnold-Chiari malformation, hydrocephalus, deformation of the head and anomalous spine, deformed feet, the conclusion of the panel of geneticists was straightforward—to terminate, a baby with those defects can't survive.... they induced labor, when I gave birth they covered my eyes, said not to look, otherwise I'd remember it for the rest of my life

Guest Don't trust doctors it's better to go to Saint Matrona, she'll help. You can also go to holy places.

Ulyana I'll never forget the day I signed the consent form to kill my own daughter.... The little girl inside me fought and grew, hands, feet all developed properly, but they said her heart was beginning to fail in those conditions, everything was hyperatrophied. They diagnosed delayed development. Said she wouldn't live. They convened a medical council.... To this day I can't forgive myself that I doubted her ability to survive.... It was as if she was showing me that she could, she was growing, but I made the decision for her. Lord I don't wish for anyone to go through that—to kill your own child.... At 10:30 a.m. they gave me sodium chloride...inserted a laminaria stick, then my stomach hurt terribly, it went on for 4 hours without stopping. Starting that morning they gave me shots 3 times a day of No-Spa with oxytomycin (I think) that same sodium chloride and something else. The contractions started around 7 p.m., after 9 p.m. the contractions started coming every 30 seconds, with them non-stop vomiting, at 1:40 a.m. I gave birth to my murdered daughter....

I'm registered at the local outpatient gynecological clinic, but all sixteen weeks I've been under the care of the V. F. Snegiryov Obstetrics and Gynecology Clinic

---

[1] Author's note: Here and throughout the text, these and other responses from participants in online chats have been taken from open sources on the internet; original spelling and punctuation have been retained.

that's on Yelansky Street, next to Bolshaya Pirogovskaya Street. I've been paying for my care there. And I'd planned to give birth there, also at my own expense. I thought it would be more reliable. During my first pregnancy, I never lost the feeling that there, inside my uterus, everything was hanging by a thread. They constantly wrote "threat of miscarriage," and I was hospitalized for some time as a precaution. Despite all that, Little Badger was born at full term, but I decided I'd be smarter the second time. The local gynecological clinic—what was that? There were lines, everyone was irritated and clueless there. Paid care would be better. Better qualified doctors, better quality equipment, and so forth. During this second pregnancy, my pulse was over one hundred and twenty, but there'd been no threats about miscarriage. Big Badger even joked that this baby had seized hold of me so tightly that there was no getting rid of him.

Now, we know that there's a way to get rid of him. If they don't die in the womb, these children are born with enormous stomachs. Their stomachs consist mainly of kidneys. And the kidneys consist of cysts. Their stomachs are so big that it hinders them from passing through the birth canal, and a caesarian section is required. Their lungs are underdeveloped because of the pressure of the kidneys and the compression connected to the absence of amniotic fluid. They can't breathe. They live from several minutes to several months on artificial respiration. They have high arterial pressure. They have "Potter facies"—not to be confused with the beloved book character. Potter syndrome is a facial deformity that comes from the lack of amniotic fluid. A flattened nose; narrow, widely spaced eyes; deformed ears.

And then, there's our daughter—she's so beautiful. She's very beautiful.

I telephone the doctor who saw me at the Snegiryov Clinic. I tell him about the giant kidneys and polycystic kidney disease. And about the fact that I may have to terminate the pregnancy.

"That's a very serious diagnosis," he says. "And termination is a very serious procedure."

"Yes, I know. What should I do? When should I come back to see you?"

"I don't see much point in coming to see me now. You should consult with perinatologists. At the Filatovskaya Hospital, for example. But in general, if the diagnosis is confirmed, then the prognosis for survival is unfavorable. I'd advise you to go as quickly as possible to the local gynecological clinic. Time is working against you now. You're well into the pregnancy. The gynecological clinic gives the authorization for termination."

"And if I get that authorization, can I terminate the pregnancy in your clinic?"

Until now, he's spoken gently and compassionately with me. After this question, something changes in his tone. It's as if I've proposed he do something dirty and perverted with me.

"No, we don't do that here. We don't deal with those things."

I call around to several clinics and maternity hospitals with good reputations, both free and paid. They don't deal with those things, either. "What things?" "You know: abortions late in a pregnancy!" "But it's for medical reasons!" "Then go to the local gynecological clinic." And I also ask if they'll oversee a pregnancy with these kinds of defects. For money. If, for example, I decide to carry the baby to term. But they don't deal with those things, either. In one of the clinics, they say, indignantly, "What's wrong with you, ma'am? How can you imagine such a thing? We have pregnant women here. Looking at you, they'll worry!"

They have pregnant women there. Preggy-weggies. There, they look after preggy-weggies and their belly-dwellers, but not any kind of pathological abomination. They control their weight and the composition of their blood and the beating of their hearts. But if something goes wrong, if the work of the primary cilia in the epithelial cells of the kidney tubules is disrupted, if the parenchyma degenerates into cysts, if the prognosis is unfavorable, if those kinds of children don't survive—then the belly-dweller turns into a fetus with a defect, into a rotting pumpkin; the preggy-weggy turns into a rat. All these clinics. With balloons, with *Your Little One* magazines, with photographs of infants, with bras for future mamas. They aren't for rats. Let the rats leave through the back door. Let the rats creep around the cellar. Those who are expecting little ones come through the front door. Future mamas come through the front door. But I'm not expecting, already I'm not expecting anyone. I'm simply a rat. And my future is outlined in the manuals of the Center for Sanitary Supervision and Disease Control.

The advantage of being a pregnant journalist over being a pregnant non-journalist lies in the fact that a pregnant journalist is able to quickly collect information, even when she's in complete despair and dripping snot. With just a couple of hours' research, I clarify that late termination of pregnancy is done for medical or social reasons in strictly specialized institutions. In the main, these institutions are obstetrical-gynecological inpatient facilities in specific hospitals. These facilities treat pregnant and non-pregnant women, including those with viral infections, with purulent-septic lesions, with inflammations of the reproductive system, with chronic genitourinary infections, after underground abortions, women who aren't properly registered to live in the city, who have incomplete pregnancy check-up records, who are homeless. Late-term abortion for social reasons happens in cases of women suffering from drug addiction, alcoholism, psychiatric disorders, women without any material means, "without anyone to feed them." Late-term abortion for medical reasons—that's my situation. A threat to the life of the mother or severe birth defects in the fetus. You can obtain a referral for such an institution only at the local gynecological clinic where you live.

In Moscow, "such an institution" is, for example, the obstetrical inpatient facility of Infectious Diseases Clinical Hospital No. 2. It's located in the Sokolinaya Gora district. If you're a man or woman who's never been expecting, you probably don't know that people love to frighten careless preggy-weggies with Sokolinaya Gora. "If you don't come for regular checkups, we won't fill out your check-up record, and you'll have to give birth in Sokolinaya Gora with the bums." During my first pregnancy, they talked to me like that at the local gynecological clinic. Although during my second pregnancy, which requires termination, they'll say something different. That at the hospital in Sokolinaya Gora there are specially trained doctors, professionals and masters of their work. That they and only they are capable of terminating a pregnancy late in the term. Real skill is required for that. Because it's a serious business. Something might suddenly go wrong. A hemorrhage. Or the need to remove the uterus.

And of course, what kind of research would it be without reading reviews and testimonials in online chat rooms? I read hundreds of them, maybe thousands. It's an entire world. These are the soldiers of the Rat King who've lost the battle. Maimed, bleeding profusely, retreating hissing and shrieking to their underground lairs...

Lyolya When on the 20th of July I underwent induced labor for medical reasons they detected Arnold-Chiari malformation in my child, I learned what PAIN is. When it's terrifying to close your eyes, when it's impossible to look at other children, you become like an open wound that continually bleeds. I was late in the pregnancy in the 26th week, they induced labor for 7 days, inserted a laminaria stick, gave me shots.... my son was alive and kicked very hard. When they punctured the amniotic sac and the waters broke, my stomach took on his shape and I could feel the heartbeat of the fetus with my hand. Then I began to lose a lot of blood, I don't know why and labor stopped completely and it was decided to perform an abortion. They cut him into pieces inside me while he was alive and extracted the pieces.

Guest mothers who do such terrible things are simple bitches....

Olga Thank God I didn't endure that horror, but I can say with certainty that a child must live for as long a time as God gives him! not as long as doctors give him. Let him live 1 hour, 1 minute, but You will know that you didn't kill him

From an article on the *Women's Doctor* site:

For termination, a dose of the hormone prostaglandin is administered, which induces contractions and the slow dilation of the cervix. This process can be very long and painful....

In late pregnancy, labor is much more often induced with the aid of mifepris-tone and an analog of prostaglandin.

Still another means of inducing birth is a saline abortion, or "flooding."[2] The fluid of the amniotic sac is pumped out using a needle, and a saline solution is introduced. In a short while, the fetus will die from chemical burns and brain hemorrhage. Over the course of the next two days, the child's dead body is ex-tracted from the woman's body....

It sometimes happens that the baby is born alive, and in that case is given an injection of potassium chloride, which causes the heart to stop.

From an article on *Allwomans.ru*:

Doctors term such a fetus "a lollipop," as the effect of the saline solution on the skin of the baby means that it becomes very thin and turns bright red. The dead fetus is extracted after 24-48 hours.

Maxim I would never in my life agree to such a thing! Some women can't have children, and yet someone can perform this kind of atrocity! These poor children, wracked with pain and dead before being born!

katya L. I'm 20 years old my pregnancy was wanted I don't drink or smoke.... defects incompatible with life spina bifida, fluid in the brain, the banana sign, bifurcation of the spine in the sacral region, and something with one foot. I lost all reason to live and was admitted to the hospital.... they gave me pills every 3 hours. From 9 a.m. until 5 p.m. the pain was un-bearable they said to use suppositories so the uterus would relax and they only gave me diarrhea finally at 9:20 p.m. they took me from the room to give birth they pierced the amniotic sac the waters broke and I gave birth to a girl (she was dead) and the placenta came out then anesthesia I don't know why. PLEASE GOD may no one else go through this I sit and read and howl my mind is broken I don't want to speak with anyone I want to die.

Olga I keep hearing this phrase: "What *I* went through," notice the stress on the word *I*. You don't want to let your "defective" baby live first of all because you don't want to experience the suffering of seeing and under-standing that the baby will die. At the same time, admittedly with diffi-culty, you agree with the decision to dissolve the baby inside you in a saline solution.... Most of all, you're sorry for *yourself*!

---

[2] As far as I know, "flooding" is not now used in Russia—at least, not in large cities. All the same, this "bogeyman" is widely discussed both online and in gynecological clinics.

Saturnina I cannot respect those who kill living children. You still want children? What kind of mother will you be?... Those who kill their own children will only get censure and shame.

For several hours, I fill my head full of this dark, obstetrical-gynecological netherworld. And even later, when it looks as if I've come up for air, I'm being dragged back all the time. Nothing in the world interests me more than these pathological reports from hell. The phrase "reading about horrors" becomes part of the everyday lexicon Big Badger and I use.

"What, are you reading about horrors again?"

"Yes."

"For what reason?"

"So I'll know."

I read about the possible consequences of "induced labor" on one's health (that's a whole different story, from infection and hemorrhage to the complete loss of the ability to have children in the future).

I read about "cleaning out," which is also called "scraping out"—both phrases are repulsive. Cleaning out takes place at the very end, under anesthesia, regardless of whether any fragments of the placenta remain in the uterus, just in case. Sometimes they "clean out" the uterus several times because they use the curette blindly, without the aid of an ultrasound, and something manages to remain behind. I'm afraid of anesthesia. I'm afraid of being scraped out. I'm afraid of the curette. I'm afraid of all these words. I don't want to be scraped and cleaned out with a sharp curette.

I read about saline abortions and lollipop infants.

I read the stories of women who've held the dead body of their belly-dweller in their arms.

I read the stories of women whose families disintegrated after an "induced birth."

I read the stories of women who never find peace.

I read the questions "What did I do to deserve this?" and "How can I live now?" and "Could the doctors have made a mistake?"

I read the comments of those who sympathize and the comments of those who make angry denunciations.

I read confessions and homilies.

I don't know why I read all this, because I already have an ocean of information. Probably, I just want to receive constant confirmation that I'm not alone. That there's a whole, huge cellar of these rats like me, and that they all squeal in pain and fear.

Trolls are confined in the cellar together with the rats. Trolls who write about infanticide and about the barrel of saline solution waiting in hell and about God, who alone decides who lives and who dies.

In general, there are two kinds of God in these chat rooms. There's the God of Punishment, the one who casts everyone in his or her turn into sodium chloride, and the Super-Duper Expert God. Super-Duper Expert God (and also his deputies— Saint Matrona and the priests) is able to correct bad ultrasound results, heal chromosomal anomalies, and disprove diagnoses.

Undoubtedly, in situations where the only hope left is a miracle, appealing to a higher power is entirely natural. Personally, I'm agnostic, but if I were a believer, if I didn't doubt that someone on high is listening to me, saying a prayer would make things easier for me. Faith in a miracle is natural. Prayer is natural. What's unnatural is when prayer and medicine, diagnosis and faith, take one another's place. When advice concerning birth defects comes from a priest. "The doctors order termination the baby has no brain how can I help my child?" "Don't listen to the doctors, go to Saint Matrona...." That's the degree of despair and derangement you have to reach.

Guest Go to the priest and ask whether to terminate the pregnancy or not.

Alfina I cried out to the whole clinic that I'd hang myself.... I'm going to kill my child and myself!... she was in pain, a lot of pain. i didn't feel her anymore.... I go to my appointment at the gynecologist and o GOD I haven't been "cleaned out," the hospital again. Being "cleaned out." tears. i just can't. just a walking corpse. then there's still a cyst, and what did I want? to kill my child and that's it? to live peacefully after that?

Mikhaylovna You're murderers, my girls. It's the same kind of murder as walking down the street towards a sick child, an old man ... and beating him to death—why should he suffer and infect others? Any alcoholic with a ton of kids is better than you. Instead of carrying your own flesh and blood—your pain—to term ... giving birth, doing everything possible to save your little one, baptizing the child or, God forbid, closing its dear eyes and committing it to the earth in a Christian manner, you'll give it up for organs and rejuvenating cream for aging ladies. It's not surprising that the nurses treat you with disdain. I'd have you sterilized. P.S. You'll end up in a barrel of saline solution. In hell.

The special ability of a journalist with a pathological pregnancy—and not, say, of an artist—is again evident when the Russian-speaking cellar full of rats isn't enough for her, and it's necessary to crawl into the English-speaking one as well to get the full picture. I crawl in....

In English-language chat rooms, of course, God is also present, but he's a little different. Not a God of Punishment and not a Super-Duper Expert God, but something like a cosy cat—or, at the very least, like a mom. He's homey, he soothes, and he displays solicitude to the best of his ability. You can even resent him or get angry that he doesn't do his job properly. In chat rooms dedicated to birth defects, you can even find separate threads like "Our relationship with God after loss." Besides God, another personage constantly appears there—the psychologist. Like something that's a given in that situation. Not as a last resort to which you run only when you've come to the end of your rope.

In general, English-language chat rooms remind one much less of a cellar. First of all, because a wonderful order reigns there: all the suffering, like all the mutations, is precisely laid out. For example, there's a popular site with the awful, soap-opera-like name of *A Heartbreaking Choice*. Along the left side of the screen runs a column listing various fetal abnormalities: anencephaly, congenital brain defects, congenital heart defects, hydrocephalus, Potter syndrome (including my situation), spina bifida, Triple X syndrome 13, Triple X syndrome 18, Triple X syndrome 21 (Downs), and so forth. You click your mouse on the one you need—you read "heartbreaking stories" on the topic. There's a massive number of sites dedicated exclusively to one particular disorder. Do you want to "talk about it"? Go to the discussion section on the site. And observe the proper rules and rituals.

The most important rule: if you are, for example, a religious fanatic, an online troll, or if you simply have your own personal opinion about the impermissibility of late-term abortion, or if it accidentally becomes clear to you that there's a direct connection between the termination of pregnancy for medical reasons and the fires of hell, then you're warned, politely, in all caps, that you shouldn't comment in the chat room. Because this is a place for women who are experiencing loss and are in pain, and you shouldn't distress them. Because they'll quickly ban you anyway— and in the best-case scenario, that's that. In the worst case, you'll end up in court for causing psychological distress. You don't want to end up in court? Create your own discussion club dedicated to the flames of hell, and enjoy yourself to your heart's content.

Not once in even a single English-language chat room did I run into a single aggressive idiot with an opinion along the lines of "mother-murderer." Not because there aren't aggressive idiots in the US, Canada, or Australia—there are no fewer of them there than here in Russia—but because there are rules.

Because "their" discussions on birth defects and the termination of pregnancy are a form of psychotherapy. And "ours" are a form of self-torture.

And about rituals. One of the obligatory rituals on the English-language sites: any personal outpouring in response to some stranger's outpouring is preceded with one simple phrase: "I'm sorry for your loss."

Perhaps, in actual fact, you don't sympathize with anyone. Maybe you're thinking only of your own sorrow. But all the same, you sit and type that simple phrase. Just so as to not feel yourself to be a rat in a cellar.

CHAPTER 5
A CHANCE

All the same, I find still another ultrasound expert—Olga Malmberg. She has a full schedule in the coming days, but on hearing the diagnosis, she says: "Come tomorrow." Her ultrasound is also expensive—even more expensive than Voyevodin's—but at the moment, the question of finances doesn't worry me at all. Money's just paper with pictures on it. We don't have any extra money left, we live in a rental apartment, so I go into the envelope marked "for December" and take the money from there. In the bottom of the red nightstand, between the contract for a script and an album of Badger's drawings, I've stored away yet another envelope—it's money for the birth. But I don't want to take money from there. It suddenly seems to me that the presence of an envelope with money for the birth somehow increases my chances that a birth will actually take place.

I take Big Badger with me to this ultrasound.

We wait a long time in the hallway of the Mother and Child private clinic; all around us are preggy-weggies to one degree or another full of life, and also "IVF ladies"—women who've come for in vitro fertilization procedures. An artificial Christmas tree is wound around with tinsel. A carnival atmosphere. On the wall is a large plasma screen, and I goggle at it so as not to look at anyone's stomach. On TV, I see some kind of jolly guy, also with a stomach, cooking something unbearably rich, rosy, and soft, which he then submits to the judgment of some ladies, and they give him a saucepan for it, and they're all very happy...

"Diffuse enlargement of the kidney, a hyperechogenic structure, with multiple cysts..." Olga Malmberg looks sadly at the screen—it seems genuine—and dictates to her assistant. "Be patient, folks," that's directed at us. "I'll finish the examination now, and we'll discuss everything... So, the placenta... three vessels... a normal amount of amniotic fluid... the cerebellum... The heartbeat... The feet... The baby's sex... a boy..."

I lie there with my eyes screwed shut. Her voice, describing the boy in my stomach in great detail, reaches me through the thud of my own heart. That voice doesn't say anything new, nothing I wouldn't have heard in the previous ultrasounds, but it sounds calm and also sad, and it says, "Be patient" and it calls me "sweetie" and my baby a baby and not a fetus, and it calls Badger and me "folks," and it says, "I'm very sorry..." It's simply a good, human voice, not more and not less. Just right for me to find the strength in myself to open my eyes and get dressed when everything's done.

"Well, folks, I've looked at everything," says Olga Malmberg. "Your little one has bilateral multicystic dysplastic kidney. I'm very sorry. I don't see any other birth defects. These children..."

"... don't survive don't survive don't survive" thrums in my head.

"... must undergo hemodialysis immediately after birth, if they manage to survive. Later, they need an artificial kidney," she adds.

"Do you mean there's a chance he'll survive?"

"It's a very small chance," Malmberg answers. "If it's an isolated defect and not part of some kind of chromosomal deformation. If the function of just one of his kidneys is preserved to some degree. All of this will be clear in two weeks. We'll see if any other defects appear. If there's amniotic fluid. In the absence of amniotic fluid, there's no chance. Then, there'll be compression, his lungs won't develop... The baby won't die from kidney failure—he simply won't be able to breathe. If the function of just one kidney is preserved, the amniotic fluid will be retained, and it's possible to try to save the baby. Although with this kind of birth defect, you have the right to terminate the pregnancy in any case. It's your decision."

"I don't want to terminate the pregnancy," I say.

"We don't want to," echoes Big Badger, in a dull voice.

She nods: "Then let's simply try to be calm and wait two weeks and then repeat the ultrasound. Your gestational period then will be eighteen or nineteen weeks. It's not too late for termination if a shortage of amniotic fluid is revealed... It's hard, I understand. It's hard to wait. And the chance is very small, folks."

"Is there anything I can do to retain the amniotic fluid?" I ask. "Anything?"

I'm prepared to drink water by the cup, by the liter. Or they can give it to me through an IV drip. Maybe then even a little of it will reach him?...

"You can't do anything," she says simply. "Just wait. I hope you get lucky."

We don't get lucky. But for those two weeks of hope and postponement that she gave us, I'm grateful to Olga Malmberg to this day.

During those two weeks, I somehow wrote up my story about the troubled family with many children and the social service authorities (the children, by the way, remained with the mother).

During those two weeks, I was able to say dozens, hundreds of times to my own unborn baby: Stay with us. Please, stay with us, stay with us. We'll love you. We'll play with you. You'll like it. Don't go. Don't forsake us.

During those two weeks, I was able to say dozens, hundreds of times to the child I already have that none of this is her fault. It's paradoxical, but my eight-year-old daughter thought she was responsible for what happened. "Is it all because of me?" "Is it because I asked you to give me a sister or brother?" "Is it because I caught a cold and brought infection into the house?"

During those two weeks, I was able to study and reckon with all the possibilities, the variables. How and where to save the baby if the amniotic fluid remained. How and where to terminate the pregnancy if the fluid was gone. For the most part, the two main variants of termination were the gynecological ward of an isolation hospital here in Russia (through the local gynecological clinic) or a good clinic that isn't squeamish about "doing that kind of thing" abroad. According to Russian law, no clinic—other than one that specializes, like the one in Sokolinaya Gora—has the right to perform a late-term abortion for medical reasons: not a paid one, not a free one.

Those two weeks were simply my time, time won, time that couldn't be taken away from me even by the women working in the local gynecological clinic. Without that time and that hope, I'd probably have surrendered and done everything they wanted—immediately, obediently, without any alternative. It's possible that wonderful specialists really do work at the Moscow isolation clinic, I don't know anything about that. It's just that during those two weeks, I finally understood that I should have the right to choose where and how I wanted to terminate the pregnancy: with the patients in isolation or not, with anesthesia or without, in the presence of my husband or alone. The isolation hospital offered a "quick and dirty" package of services: hospitalization from ten to fourteen days, artificially induced birth without anesthesia, cutterage, a course of antibiotics, visits from relatives—during strictly controlled hours.

Through friends and acquaintances living abroad, I inquired at several foreign clinics. In Hungary, France, and somewhere else they expressed sympathy and refused—they don't terminate pregnancy in the later stages for foreigners without a residence permit. By the way, the Hungarian doctor mentioned that "saline abortions" haven't been used there since the 1970s and that they use the most merciful means possible. They were prepared to take me in Israel, but the affair required an enormous sum of money and promised a mass of bureaucratic obstacles and delays. The most practical option turned out to be the clinic at Charité-Universitätsmedizin in Berlin, with which my friend Natasha, who'd lived in Germany for a long time, agreed in advance. However, termination at Charité wasn't cheap, either—especially as they quoted only an approximate sum of five thousand euros and were prepared to name a final sum only after an examination and ultrasound. Considering that we also needed money for tickets, a rental apartment in Berlin, and associated expenses, there wasn't even a quarter of what we needed in our envelope "for the birth," and the whole undertaking seemed, to put it gently, doubtful.

We began collecting money from friends and acquaintances but all the same, in parallel, just in case we didn't collect enough money or something went wrong with the visas, I went to the local gynecological clinic that the luminary of science had so urgently recommended to me.

CHAPTER 6
YOU'LL HAVE OTHERS

"No men allowed," the gloomy, muscle-bound man in the grey sweater bars our way. He's a guard. He guards the district gynecological clinic in Khamovniki. From men.

"This is my husband," I say.

"No men allowed," the guard repeats, in a bored voice. "Those are the rules."

"Please let me in," says my husband. It seems he sincerely believes it's possible to explain things to the gloomy man in the mouse-colored sweater. "We have a really serious situation. Truly serious. We need to speak with the doctor together."

"No men are allowed here, mister," the guard plants his feet widely apart, as if to demonstrate that no power in the world will disturb him from faithfully executing his duties. "This is a women's institution. Let the woman go alone. While you wait, have a seat here, on the bench."

We give up. My husband sits on the bench, and I go alone. I climb to the second floor and sit on a different bench—across from the doctor's office—in an endless line of women. Those are the rules. No men allowed. Men have nothing to do with this. No men allowed to come close to women's institutions, to women's illnesses and woes. That's how the people who devised those rules think. That's how the women in the line think themselves. That's how the doctor in the clinic thinks. That's how my mother thinks. When she found out that I wanted Sasha to be next to me at the "induced birth," she was horrified:

"You want to lose your husband, too, do you? Why does he need to see that nightmare? Men disappear after that kind of thing!"

The obstetrician-gynecologist serving my microdistrict is, in essence, a good woman. Hearing about polycystic kidney disease, it seems she sympathizes with me absolutely sincerely—and she even tries to comfort me, as best she can. She unleashes a flood of folk wisdom on me, most of which I've already encountered in chat rooms. She says:

"Don't cry, you're still young, you'll have another one, a healthy one."

She says:

"You'll terminate now, and in a year, you'll be pregnant again, you won't be struck by bad luck twice."

She says:

"God tests us according to our strength. If he gave this burden to you, it means that you can bear it."

Then, she says I have to immediately, immediately go through a medical council to receive permission for termination and check into the specialized hospital. She looks for my pregnancy check-up record and can't find it, there is no record. That's entirely my fault—I really had registered the pregnancy at eight weeks, but I didn't go to the clinic after that, preferring "those private doctors" to her and, naturally, during that period my record "disappeared"—but she forgives me. Now, we'll quickly set up a new one for me. Because I have to immediately, immediately be registered anew.

"So, look, this is what we'll do. You go downstairs now to the registration desk and they'll set up a new check-up record for you. Then you come back here, I'll register you again and give you a medical referral, with it, you visit the doctors in the district polyclinic: the therapist, dental surgeon, cardiologist—because your pulse is simply racing!—the otolaryngologist, the optician... They have to fill out this checklist. Bring it back here. Otherwise—without this checklist—I can't hand you the check-up record. And your husband also has to go and get an x-ray of his lungs. Then we can convene the council—and..."

"I still haven't decided," I say, quietly.

"What haven't you decided?"

"Whether I'm going to terminate this pregnancy. They told me that if there's any amniotic fluid left in two weeks, then there's a chance..."

"What are you talking about?" barks the good woman, but immediately softens. As before, she's sorry for me. She looks at me as if I'm crazy. As if I'm an insane Ophelia who plaits daisies in her tangled hair, singing to herself, instead of running immediately to the district polyclinic with the checklist. "She hasn't decided!... She has a chance!... Do you even understand what will happen to your life if you have this child? He'll be completely disabled, very seriously disabled, a freak! And you'll be all alone with him! Don't you know husbands don't stick around long with these kinds of children! Don't even think about it. Later, you'll have a healthy one. So, now, off you go to registration..."

"But all the same, if the amniotic fluid remains, I plan to have this child. It'll be clear in two weeks."

"If the fluid remains! Two weeks! You don't have two weeks! The clock is ticking! In two weeks, he'll probably already weigh five hundred grams! And when they weigh five hundred grams, by law the doctors have to save them! Do you understand? Say you have him—they'll torment him, resuscitate him, and all the same, he won't be able to survive! Do you need all that?"

"And if he weighs less than five hundred grams?" unexpectedly inquires that other businesslike and collected me. "Then what?"

"Then he'll be born dead," says the good woman. "And now, go to the first floor to the registration desk and set up your check-up record."

I go to the registration desk, icy and somehow not fully whole—like a piece of wood that snaps in frost. Opposite the registration desk, my husband sits on the bench.

"Well?" he leaps up.

"I have to set up a check-up record," I say, stupidly.

The benevolent old lady behind the registration desk enters my information into the computer.

"How long have you been pregnant?"

"Sixteen weeks."

She presents me with some kind of paper, with which I have to go back upstairs to the gynecologist's office, and a gift pack. In it is a sample of cream for stretch marks, an advertising brochure for the maternity hospital, and a disposable diaper.

I look at the disposable diaper. I look at it a long time. So long that the wooden and businesslike me manages to get bored and disappears somewhere. And the overwhelmed and spineless me begins to cry. And to say to Big Badger:

"I don't want to kill him...! I want to have him and put this diaper on him!..."

The baby inside me shudders slightly—like a moth caught in your hand.

"Ma'am, we have pregnant women here!" says some woman in a white lab coat, who up until now has been silently observing us, reproachfully. "And look how you're carrying on!..."

Big Badger stands between her and me, and he hugs me. He strokes my head. And he whispers:

"Let's get out of here..."

For that, he sat there on the bench two hours. So he could hug me and take me away from that women's hell into the cold, autumn darkness, where people of both sexes can go.

That same evening my parents, who until now thought the idea of running away to Charité was absurd, call and say they can give us a large part of the necessary sum. They've also read the stories in the chat rooms about late termination of pregnancy. Friends promise to lend the rest of the money. We buy airplane tickets online. By some astonishing coincidence, the cheapest turn out to be for that same day when we have the ultrasound scheduled with Malmberg. We decide what to do. We'll take our suitcases to the ultrasound. If the amniotic fluid remains, we'll simply lose the cost of the tickets. If there's no fluid, we'll go straight from the clinic to the airport. Little Badger will stay with my parents.

"Unfortunately, folks, almost no amniotic fluid remains."

We go to the airport through a slush of snow and mud.

We sit on the plane. In the window is dark, icy emptiness. Usually, I'm very scared of flying, but I'm not afraid now. It doesn't matter to me whether the airplane crashes or not.

I've already crashed.

CHAPTER 7
VERDICT IN GERMAN

In the clinic at Berlin's Charité-Universitätsmedizin, I'm seen by Professor Kalache, a German luminary of ultrasound diagnostics who specializes in intrauterine birth defects. We speak English; just in case we need to translate anything from German, my friend Natasha accompanies us.

The first thing Dr. Kalache says to me when we enter his office is:

"I'm so sorry you've come to our clinic for such a sad reason."

He guides the probe over my stomach, and my son's face appears on a big screen. He's sucking one of his fingers. Will the German luminary suddenly refute the diagnosis now? Or, no, he'll say the diagnosis is mostly correct, but they're able to treat such things in the clinic...

"Unfortunately, I can only confirm the diagnosis given to you in Moscow. This is infantile polycystic kidney disease—or else bilateral multicystic dysplastic kidney. There's no amniotic fluid. In any case, the prognosis for life is unfavorable. I'm really very sorry. This little baby has no chance."

He calls him a "baby." In the ultrasound report, in the postmortem protocol, my son will be called a "fetus." But in spoken conversations, addressing me and my husband, the Charité employees only use the word "baby." Because they've conducted psychological research here. No one, no one in the world knows if a fetus has a soul. But on the other hand, according to the research, it's known for certain that it's easier for a woman when her doomed fetus is called a "baby" and not a "fetus." They don't refuse to give the child human, child-like characteristics.

Constantly hearing that word, "baby," my husband also quickly begins to call our baby a baby. Not because I insist on it—it's simply automatic...

"The baby's head is located downwards. If you don't mind, I'd like to look at the brain transvaginally," says Dr. Kalache. "The thing is, these alterations in the kidney might be an isolated defect or part of some kind of syndrome. In that case, we'll also see an alteration in the brain. Please, take off your clothes below the waist. You don't object to the presence of your husband and your friend during this part of the exam? Maybe you'd like them to leave?"

"Let them stay." I recall Professor Demidov and his fifteen students.

Dr. Kalache covers me with a disposable sheet so my naked body won't be visible and inserts the probe into my vagina.

"The brain is developing normally," he concludes. "Please, get dressed. Now, I'll tell you what you can do next and what kind of choice you have."

And he tells us. Once more, pay attention. Professor Kalache—one of the most famous specialists on fetal pathology in Germany—doesn't send me to the local gynecological clinic, to an assistant, or anywhere else, but simply tells us himself, calmly and in detail, what to do now and how.

The "plan of action" in our case is clear enough. The professor will give me a paper with the ultrasound results, the diagnosis, and a special postscript at the end: "At the woman's request, termination of this particular pregnancy may be performed." No additional permissions, checklists, or medical councils for termination are necessary for me, a foreigner, or for any German woman—the professor's diagnosis in and of itself is sufficient grounds. Furthermore, by law, a woman is given three days to consider whether to terminate the pregnancy or carry it to term. Moreover, it's three days not in the sense that she can't think longer than that, but the exact opposite: she's required to think not *less* than three days. During those three days, she must also make an obligatory visit to a psychologist, ideally together with her partner. Moreover, the responsibility for that visit lies with the doctor—the doctor might even be fired if it becomes clear that he didn't recommend that the woman make an appointment with the psychologist and, in the case of her refusal, insist on it. Several psychologists—"specialists in loss"—work with the maternity ward of the clinic, and the appointment is free. But neither the psychologists nor the medical staff have the right to exert moral pressure or in any way urge the woman and the family towards one outcome or the other. At the end of the three days, the woman communicates her decision to the clinic.

"I came here specifically in order to terminate the pregnancy if the diagnosis was confirmed," I say. "I don't need to think about it for three days, and I don't need a psychologist, either. In Russia, doctors don't want to take on this kind of pregnancy, even if I decide to carry it to term."

"All the same, you have three days," says the doctor. "You don't have to think about it if you don't want to. But I'd very strongly recommend that you and your husband make an appointment with the psychologist. It's free. Nothing worse can come from it. On the other hand, it might make things easier."

"Are you recommending the psychologist to me because it's required?"

"For German women, yes. But you, as a foreign patient, aren't required to go to the psychologist. I suggest this because it seems to me that you need to do it."

"And if I were German... and chose to prolong the pregnancy... what would happen then?"

"You'd be treated like any other pregnant woman. It's possible that you'd undergo a caesarian section if, at the time of birth, the size of the baby's stomach is too big from the enlarged kidneys and might damage the birth canal."

"Do you have any statistics... what do women ordinarily decide in these situations?"

"The majority carry the pregnancy to term."

"Honestly?!"

"Yes. It's really more natural. Both psychologically and physically."

"But, really... if the baby is doomed?..."

"I have an uncle," says Professor Kalache. "He's in the last stage of cancer. He's doomed. But no one will kill him before his time. He'll die when his time comes."

Unexpectedly for me, I suddenly feel a sharp desire to carry this pregnancy to term, in spite of everything. So he can live as much as possible, if only in my uterus. I'm supposed to give birth in May. Maybe we'll find some way to stay in Germany until May?...

"And... then? This baby... They'll try to save him?"

"It's better for you to speak with the neonatologist about that," answers Kalache. "Would you like me to arrange a consultation with our neonatologist for you?"

"Yes. How much will that consultation cost?"

"I... don't know," flounders the professor. "We don't have a particular price list. For German patients, that's all covered by insurance."

For several seconds, he ponders something tensely, then his face clears:

"I think our neonatologist will be pleased to consult with you for free."

Before we leave, I ask the last question. I'm not planning to ask it, but it somehow pops out of my mouth, all by itself:

"Is there any chance, even the minutest possibility, that you've made a mistake in the diagnosis?"

Dr. Kalache answers me in the same words of that very first ultrasound doctor, the one who wasn't an expert. He says:

"I'm not the Lord God."

He says he's a man, and that he makes mistakes.

And I understand that he's absolutely certain of his diagnosis.

CHAPTER 8
YOU CAN SING HIM A SONG

The neonatologist is a young frau with a chestnut-colored bob and tender, olive eyes. Like Dr. Kalache, she expresses sympathy to me and extends her hand in greeting. Here, it's expected that doctors will shake your hand.

Just in case, Natasha is with us—but the conversation again takes place in English. The neonatologist says she's seen the results of my ultrasound. She's very sorry but she, like Dr. Kalache, thinks our baby has no chance of survival. She doesn't know that we came from Moscow specifically for a termination, and it seems she thinks we live in Berlin. Therefore, she announces that if we decide to prolong the pregnancy, she and her assistants will be present at the birth in order to assist the newborn, however, in our case it will simply be a formality.

"You have the right to demand resuscitation, but we don't see any sense in that. There are less serious cases of this pathology—but your case is very serious. Eighteen weeks—and already there's absolutely no amniotic fluid. That means that the baby's lungs won't develop. We've seen many such newborns. Unfortunately, they...."

... don't survive... don't survive...

"... don't survive. They perish either at birth, or a few minutes after or, at a maximum, a few hours after birth—regardless of whether we try to save them or not."

"And therefore, you think it's right to not even try to save them?!"

Her olive eyes open wide in surprise:

"If it's impossible in any case to save the baby, why take the child away from the parents to be tortured with all kinds of tubes and a ventilator? Not long ago, we had a sad case here. The baby was born with the same kind of kidney defect as yours. The child couldn't breathe. His parents insisted on resuscitation. We fulfilled their request—but the ventilator didn't help the child breathe, it simply..." Here, she hesitates.

The neonatologist doesn't know how to say something in English. She addresses Natasha in German and quickly explains something. Natasha's face changes:

"The ventilator... tore the baby's lungs."

"I think that was wrong," the neonatologist continues, in English. "That we tortured him for no reason."

"But... how will we then... what will happen then?" mutters my husband.

"The baby is born—and we leave the family together in a separate room with the baby. We don't disturb the parents saying goodbye. You can stay in that room with the baby all day if you want, even after the baby dies. You can dress the baby however you like. Sing the baby a song. Take photos. If you're a religious believer, we can invite a member of the clergy of the corresponding faith for you."

"The baby... the baby... dies right there in the arms of the parents? Without any doctors?" I ask.

"Doctors aren't necessary in order to die."

I imagine how my baby won't be able to breathe. How he'll turn blue and die. And I'll dress him as I like, and sing him a song. *Havana sleeps, Athens sleeps, autumn flowers sleep... Dolphins sleep in the Black Sea, and whales sleep in the White Sea...*

"But that's really scary," I say to the neonatologist, for some reason. "Sitting in a room with a dead baby."

"It's more scary, probably, to give the baby to the morgue right away. Usually, a woman wants to be with her baby as long as possible."

In parting, she asks when we're going to see the psychologist.

"We don't want to see the psychologist," I say. "The psychologist can't help his lungs open."

"The psychologist isn't to help the baby, but to help you."

I smile:

"The psychologist can't help me."

No one can help me.

Chapter 9
The Choice: Those Three Terrible Days

We're renting a tourist apartment—with a kitchen, bedroom, and living room—on a quiet little street of burghers, Spenerstrasse. The owner of the apartment asks whether we're doing well and enjoying our time in Berlin. We answer politely, yes, all's well. In general, I'd have preferred to spend all these days in bed, motionless, with my face to the wall. But they don't let me do that. Every morning, Sasha lifts me out of bed and forces me to eat something. Every day, Natasha comes by and takes us to look around the city. Wreaths, lights, gingerbread cookies, Christmas trees, and mulled wine are everywhere. We tramp along the ice-covered streets, we stop in cafés and bars. I drink mulled wine because it's no longer important. Because these kinds of children don't survive. And also because I feel he likes mulled wine. When I drink mulled wine, he stirs around happily inside me. For once in his life—there in the airless dark of my uterus, from which he'll never make it out to the light and air—let him experience something pleasant.

Sometimes, I cry. But as a whole, this strange, pre-Christmas city evokes the feeling of living unreality. As if I'm the main character in a low budget, art house melodrama. As if all of this isn't really happening to me: it's just a movie.

At night, when Natasha goes home and my husband goes to sleep, the movie stops, and I tumble out of it into the brothel-like comfort of a Berlin living room. Then, I cry in earnest. And I read in chat rooms about the termination of pregnancy. And about how, after late termination of pregnancy, it's not always possible to get pregnant again, and even if you get pregnant, birth defects have a habit of recurring. And also, about how people very often get divorced after this kind of thing...

And also, all these three days, unexpectedly for me, I'm still thinking. I'm choosing whether to terminate the pregnancy or carry it to term.

I want to carry it to term. Because I don't want to kill the unfortunate Littlest Badger. Because I want to give him an extra twenty weeks of life. Because I don't want to go to the hospital. Because carrying the pregnancy to term is natural and correct from the physiological point of view. Because I'm afraid of complications. Because an abortion might go badly. Because I risk losing blood, losing my health, losing my uterus, losing the ability to have children.

I want to terminate the pregnancy. Because I don't know whether all is well with him there, inside, or whether he's suffering. Could it possibly be all right when the kidneys are five times larger than normal? I want to terminate because I'm afraid I'll go out of my mind if this situation continues for several more months. If I give birth to him and watch how he dies. And then dress him, embrace him, bury him. Buy a coffin instead of a cradle. I want to terminate because in women's institutions in Russia, where men aren't allowed, the continuation of this pregnancy will be hell, and there's no way we can stay in Germany for twenty more weeks. I want to terminate so all of this will finally be over.

I try to involve Sasha in the decision, and he obediently goes around in circles with me, weighing the pros and cons. He tries not to pressure me and says he'll accept any decision I make, but when we talk about carrying the pregnancy to term, he looks away, so I won't see the panic in his eyes.

On the morning of the third day, for some reason, clarity arrives along with the ash-colored December light trickling through the slats of the Venetian blinds. I understand that this agony must come to an end. I'll terminate the pregnancy. That's why we came here.

I say this to Sasha—and he's obviously relieved.

I ask Natasha to contact the clinic at Charité and say we've reached a decision. She calls back. She says they've promised to name a date for the termination over the course of the next few days. For their part, they ask that my husband and I make an appointment with the psychologist during that time.

I think that the psychologist would have been useful to me on the day when I couldn't find my way out of the Kulakov Research Center for Obstetrics, Gynecology, and Perinatology on Oparin Street. Or the day after that. Or even a week after that. Now, there's absolutely no point in it.

But we agree. In the end, it's the polite thing to do. And even interesting, in its own way.

Chapter 10
The Psychologist from Outer Space

The psychologist—a forty-year-old woman from Holland who'd moved to Berlin in her youth—almost immediately confirms that I'm right:

"I see you've already lived through the most difficult stage during which my help might have been most useful. Did a psychologist help you in Russia?"

I begin to giggle.

"Did I say something wrong?"

I recall Professor Demidov, his fifteen students, and myself with without any underwear. I recall the recommendation to go to the local gynecological clinic. I recall the security guard in the mouse-colored sweater. And the lady at the clinic who suggests that I "have another one," who promises bad luck won't strike twice, and who demands that I immediately, immediately run quickly to the district poly-clinic with a checklist. The optician, the dental surgeon, the otolaryngologist.

"No, no psychologist helped me in Russia."

"You refused their services?"

"I wasn't offered their services."

"Very strange," the woman from Holland looks at me in disbelief. "I'm really surprised. It's standard practice!"

"Not for us," says my husband.

She nods, with an understanding look. It's not standard on Mars, either, what is there to say? Extraterrestrials have their own traditions.

"Now, I'll tell you how the termination procedure will go," she informs us. "It's important that you know several details in advance and prepare for them. It'll be easier that way. Guided by ultrasound, they'll probably give you a special shot through the abdominal wall and the uterine wall before the start of labor."

"For what purpose?"

"For the baby. For humane reasons."

I suddenly understand what she has in mind, and I freeze. "Freezing in fear"— that's a stupid cliché, but in this case, you can't find a more precise phrase. I freeze in fear. And the baby begins to fidget nervously there, in the depths, behind the abdominal wall and the uterine wall.

"What is this injection?"

"Poison," she answers calmly. "It acts in an instant. It won't affect your body. Because of it, the baby won't suffer at all during birth. And besides… at this stage of your pregnancy, there's a very small chance, but all the same a possibility, that without the shot he'll be born alive. I see it's difficult for you to hear this. But this injection saves the baby from suffering. And there are several other things that are better for you to know beforehand."

She says I'll be given the choice to receive the baby's body without an autopsy, to receive it after an autopsy, or not receive it at all. She advises us in any case to agree to an autopsy because it will help confirm or clarify the diagnosis and determine how to handle my pregnancies in future. At this stage of our conversation, the other calm and composed me luckily fills in for the me who, in her horror, has lost the gift of speech; therefore, I agree with the psychologist completely calmly: yes, it makes sense to conduct an autopsy, without question.

"Give it some thought, whether you want to receive the body—or whether you want to leave it at the hospital."

I imagine a macabre picture. So, we carry this little body from Berlin to Moscow, across the border. We pack it carefully. What have you got there in the suitcase, hey, ma'am?… That looks like a little baby?… According to our rules, it's forbidden to carry little ones in a suitcase…

"We can't really take him with us," says my husband. "What will happen to him if we leave him in the hospital?"

"They'll bury him," answers the psychologist. "You don't have to pay for that, there's money allocated in the budget. But… there's one detail. It will be a communal grave. They bury these little ones once every few months, together, in a single coffin. There will be a member of the clergy. Does it matter to you if a member of the clergy is present?"

"No."

"Well, in any case, one will be there. Two weeks before the funeral, you'll be notified about the exact date and time. You may come and participate in the ceremony, if you like."

"In a single coffin," I repeat, mechanically.

She nods:

"When I first found out about it, I was horrified myself. But later, I thought: what if it's better for them that way, for these children? Not so frightening? They aren't alone there… I'm agnostic, and I don't know if there's life after death or what kind it might be. But I thought: if, after all, there's something there, perhaps these children stick together. Maybe there they, well, you know… play together?"

I don't know if she said that sincerely, or whether it was a trained response from a professional, but later I recalled her words many times, no matter how nonsensical they seemed, and they always comforted me. They comfort me even now.

Maybe they play together there.

They aren't alone there.

"Do you have other children?" asks the psychologist.

"Yes, a daughter."

"How old is she?"

"Eight."

"Does she know what's happening?"

"Yes."

"When you return home, she'll ask you questions. About how it was."

"Yes, I know. What's the right way to answer? I don't want to lie to her."

"You don't need to lie. Spare her the heartrending details—but tell her the truth. Just one thing... don't say you chose between terminating the pregnancy and carrying it to term. Say simply that the baby couldn't live—especially because in your case, it's the absolute truth, as opposed to, say, a situation when a woman decides to terminate a pregnancy because of Down's Syndrome. Be that as it may, if a child knows that there was some kind of choice, she'll start to feel she's in danger herself. For example, she may feel she can't get sick now—or she'll be next..."

She glances over the bookshelf behind her:

"Usually, I recommend some kind of literature on the subject—but, unfortunately, everything I have is in German... In Russia, there are probably books about how to recover from the loss of a pregnancy in the later stages."

"There are no such books in Russia," I answer. "At least, I haven't found any."

I look at the bookshelf—and at that moment, the thought flashes through my brain that I myself must write "such a book" in Russian. I immediately sweep that thought aside as blasphemous. We have a tragedy here. It's not the time for books.

"I'm very sorry," she says, "that there's no helpful literature. But in any case, when you return to Moscow after the termination, it's absolutely necessary for you to go to group therapy sessions with women who, like you, have lost a baby late in pregnancy. For at least six months. It's very important to share your feelings and experience."

With difficulty, I control an idiotic giggle, entirely inappropriate for such a situation:

"There are no group therapy sessions with such women."

"Well... but it's standard practice! Probably, you just aren't aware of them. Normally, such groups are found through maternity or gynecological clinics..."

I silently shake my head. She tries to somehow comprehend this. Martians, what can you do?

At the end, already seeing us to the exit, she says:

"It's absolutely necessary to look at him."

"At whom?"

"At the baby. When he's born."

"Whatever for?"

"To say goodbye. So you don't feel guilty."

To look at the outcome of an abortion so I don't feel guilty. No, it's more likely that *they* are the Martians.

"Not for anything," I say to her. "It's very scary. If I look at him, he'll appear in my nightmares for the rest of my life."

"No, he won't." She turns to Sasha. "You're also planning not to look at him?"

"I...don't know. I haven't thought about it. What's the point?"

"To say goodbye," she repeats. "It's your baby, after all. If you don't look at him, you'll be very sorry."

We go out onto the street, towards the Christmas lights and wreaths. Towards the window displays with figurines of the Magi, the Virgin Mary, and the baby Jesus. We walk, and I keep repeating that I won't, I don't want to, I won't look at the baby.

"Don't worry, no one will force you to," says Sasha.

"And you—are you going to look at him?"

"Maybe," he considers the tiny figure of the baby in the manger behind the window glass. "I haven't decided yet."

Chapter 11
Invitation to an Execution

At last, they set the date for my hospitalization. On the day we arrive at the Charité clinic, my "gestational period" is twenty weeks. That's exactly the midpoint of pregnancy. The "equator," as they say. On the preggy-weggy sites, it's considered normal to "relax, be calm, enjoy the pregnancy, and look forward to meeting the baby" after this point.

But my equator is the finishing line. Everything ends here. There won't be any meeting.

All three of us come—I, my husband, and Natasha. In the clinic vestibule, we look for the machine that sells disposable shoe covers—we don't find it. We go up to the maternity ward in our boots, a wet trail stretching out along the floor behind us. Photographs of fat-cheeked babies hang on the corridor walls. From behind closed doors, children's cries reach us. I try not to look at the walls and not to hear any sounds. I look at my feet. I try to think only about the fact that I'm not wearing shoe covers, which is unsanitary. The first thing I say to the employee in the waiting room is:

"Excuse me, our shoes are dirty. We couldn't figure out where to buy..."

"What's the problem?" the employee is amazed. "We maintain a sterile environment only in intensive care. You can wear ordinary shoes and clothes here."

They lead us to my prenatal room. It's designed for two, but they promise me no other woman in childbirth will join me: "That would be unethical." The space is quite large: there are two convertible beds (in case it's necessary to turn them into birthing chairs), behind each bed is some kind of complicated apparatus with numerous cords and lights, a table and chairs, an electric tea kettle, a shower and toilet. In the corner is a changing table. They quickly take off the top of it, and it turns into an ordinary chest of drawers. On the wall is a call button for the midwife.

They tell us that until eleven p.m., anyone we like can be in my room, but that guests are supposed to leave at night.

"Does my husband have to leave, too?"

"Yes, your husband, too. At the very least, for tonight. Today, you'll be given a pill that prepares you for birth, but the birth itself is unlikely to happen before tomorrow. However, if it suddenly starts tonight, we'll call your husband so he can come immediately. Don't worry, he'll be present at the birth."

At the thought that I have to spend the night alone in this maternity room with convertible beds and a changing table pretending to be a chest of drawers, I become so miserable that I want to whimper. Nights are generally harder for me than days. At night, I lie on my side because sleeping on your stomach at twenty weeks is uncomfortable (or not really so uncomfortable—am I simply instinctively afraid I'll crush the baby?), and embrace my stomach with one hand (because where else can that hand go?), and I feel how he shudders there, in the darkness, and I also lie in the darkness, the darkness inside and outside of me, he and I together, as if under water, as if under the earth, he and I together, as if in a single grave. And I know all that will repeat itself tonight. I'll lie on my side so he's comfortable. Yes, I plan to get rid of him tomorrow—but today, I mustn't crush him. Tonight, he must be comfortable with me.

"What time can my husband come back tomorrow?" I ask the nurse, and I repeat to myself that I might not sleep, I just might not sleep, not sleep all night, until he arrives...

"Tonight, you must get a good night's rest." It's as if the nurse reads my thoughts. "Is it really very important that your husband stay with you?"

"Yes."

"Then, let him stay. If you want, we can move the beds so you can sleep together," she indicates with her eyes the second, empty convertible bed. "But your friend really can't stay the night. And we won't feed your husband."

"I don't plan to stay," says Natasha.

"You don't need to feed me," says my husband.

"You have to eat well," the nurse informs my husband. "You should go to a café. And you, too," she turns to me. "Now, you'll talk with the doctors, get your pill—and then go, relax. There are a lot of pleasant cafés around here."

It's hard to say what amazes me more—the suggestion to move the beds so that we can sleep together, or the suggestion to go to a café and relax.

"Um... Can we really go to a café?" my husband clarifies.

"Why not?" The nurse is surprised.

"Well, this is a hospital."

"What does that matter? We don't have any procedures scheduled today." Her sincere lack of understanding shows on her face.

"And when do we have to return?"

"Whenever you want."

"What I mean is: how late will they admit us tonight?"

"This is a hospital, not a jail. They'll let you in round the clock. Oh, and if you like to read, we have a library. You can choose any book in English. Some kind of detective novel. To distract you."

When she leaves, my husband asks:

"So, are we really going to a café?"

"I don't know," I say.

"Since they allow it, that means we should go," Natasha laughs. In general, she laughs often. She has a nice laugh.

"All right, let's go." For those happy few seconds, I suddenly forget why I'm here. Why all three of us are here. It's as if we're at Young Pioneer camp in the break between sessions. Two girls and one boy. Rest time is cancelled, we can jump on the mattresses with the iron box springs and even leave the campground.

If you terminate a pregnancy in the later stages in Russia, you stay in the hospital for a minimum of a week, more often, two. And no one, not your husband, not your mama, not your sister, not your friend—no one can be with you at night. And barely even during the day. Not for any money. And of course, no one suggests that you go to a café—that wouldn't even enter your head. If you've come to the hospital to kill your unborn child, then it's your duty to suffer. Both physically and morally. The rearranged beds, café visits, psychologists, detective novels in English, the various ways of easing your soul's pain, if only for a short time—that's all the devil's work, just like an epidural. That's how the nurses in Russia think. That's how the doctors think. That's how the clerks think. That's how the ladies on social media think. And the most interesting thing is: that's how even I think. Rather, it's not that I think that—but I feel it. The prospect of moving hospital beds bothers me. And the café as well, and the epidural. And the library. Won't that be too comfortable? Won't that be utterly despicable towards the one who they're ridding me of here?...

But here, people don't think that way. Here, they're accustomed to taking away pain—both spiritual and physical—by all means possible. And the next day when, during the birth, I try to refuse the epidural, at first the doctor will say to me that the epidural is automatically included in the cost and it's not necessary to pay extra for it, and when I answer that this has nothing to do with money, he'll say the phrase that for him is simply commonplace, but for me is a revelation: *There's no reason you should be in pain.*

Actually, it's precisely this phrase, said automatically, as a matter of course, having nothing to do with the quality of the medicine or of paid or free service, that constitutes the main difference between the Charité clinic and the isolation hospital in Sokolinaya Gora. Between all the clinics of Europe and all the hospitals of Russia. Between all the nurses, doctors, clerks, ladies and gentlemen of Europe and Russia. Just that some believe there's no reason to endure pain. And others believe pain is the norm...

Just as we're moving the beds, the doctor enters the room—a middle-aged Turk, or else an Iranian, who resembles a sad spaniel. As is customary, he greets me with a handshake, asks questions (mainly about how my first birth went), fills out some papers. He informs us that he won't be present during the birth, that only a midwife will be there.

"How can that be—just a midwife?" I'm frightened.

"If anything goes wrong, of course, I'll come," he says. "But the midwife delivers normal, uncomplicated births, that's the usual practice."

"But this really won't be a normal birth," I say. "There are no normal births at twenty weeks."

"Unfortunately, you won't have a living baby after this birth," he says. "But from the physiological point of view, your birth most likely won't differ from the most ordinary one. Especially as it's not your first birth."

"But... if I start to hemorrhage?"

"Then we'll stop it."

"And if the placenta doesn't fully detach? At this stage, it really might not all be expelled."

"Are you a doctor?"

"No. I just read about it."

"Yes, that danger exists," he nods. "It does happen in these situations. At this stage, it sometimes happens that the cervix dilates—and everything comes out immediately, both the baby and the whole placenta. Then we don't interfere with the natural process. But a fragment of the placenta can remain inside. In that case, we perform... some surgery."

Some surgery—that's what they call it. Anything is better than "cleaning" and "scraping out." I don't want to be scraped out and cleaned. But "some surgery"—that's something abstract.

"In Russia they do 'some surgery' in any case at this stage of pregnancy."

"For what reason?" He's surprised. "That's harmful to a woman's health."

"To guarantee. That nothing remains inside."

"There's the ultrasound to guarantee that," he sighs sadly, and his eyes look exactly like a spaniel's. He's a specialist who delivers babies. It seems he's sincerely sorry that this time he won't deliver anyone. That the baby won't live.

After the attending physician, the anesthesiologist arrives—a tall, handsome Aryan with clear, indifferent eyes, a grown-up Kai from "The Snow Queen." He also fills out a form (whether I have allergies, heart ailments, and so forth) and explains what the epidural is for, and general anesthesia, as well (in case "anything goes wrong"). He shows me a picture illustrating intubation of the trachea. In parting, he squeezes my hand—a short, mechanical movement—and expresses his sympathy ("I'm sorry we're meeting under such sad circumstances"). It doesn't matter to him, and he doesn't hide that. His specialty—making people unconscious for a short while—suits him.

Following the anesthesiologist is a representative of the Protestant faith community—a spare, sharp-nosed lady in a stern, dark dress, who looks like a skinny crow. She smells strongly of feminine perfume and something musty, she has icy and very powerful fingers, she makes a sad face and shakes my hand for a long time, it's irritating. Finally, she asks if we need any special ritual services for "the poor baby" and if we need a member of the clergy and, on learning that we don't, again seizes hold of my hand for a long time.

The attending midwife arrives last. She brings the pill. The one that should "prepare me for birth" (mifepristone, as I find out later from reading the medical bill). It's just a little white pill, most ordinary, absolutely innocent to look at. I'll swallow it—and it will start to kill my baby...

"This pill... how does it work?"

"It uses hormones. It tricks your body. It forces your body to believe that the time for birth has arrived."

"But it won't kill the baby?"

"No. It won't kill the baby. For that, there's a special shot."

"But the shot—that's not today? Tomorrow?"

"The shot is tomorrow," nods the midwife. "Today is just this pill."

For some reason, I feel easier. The shot isn't today. Today's just the pill, and the pill won't kill him.

I take the pill in my hand. My hands shake.

"Is it okay for me not to take it now, but in fifteen minutes?"

"That's fine," she answers. "But you must come to the staff room and take the pill in front of me. I'm responsible for that."

I note the time and sit with the pill in my hand. It won't kill him. The pill won't kill him. My baby will be with me until tomorrow. He'll move around. I'll take the pill, but he'll still move around. We'll go to the café, and I'll drink something sweet, he likes sweet things, hot chocolate or mulled wine...

After fifteen minutes, I go to the staff room. I take the pill with water. The midwife makes a note in my chart.

Then, we go to a café, and I drink mulled wine. The baby moves around. He likes sweet things, he's fine. He doesn't know that this is—farewell.

Please let him be fine. Don't let him be in pain.

Chapter 12
Bye-Bye

For physiological reasons—the shape and location of the uterus—it's impossible to perform a caesarian section during the second trimester. That is, it's impossible to surgically terminate a pregnancy under general anesthesia. It's true that there is such a thing as a "small caesarian," which is when the uterus is accessed and perforated not through the abdominal cavity but through the vagina and labia, but that method has a high probability of ensuring infertility for the rest of one's life—they resort to it only in the case of extreme necessity, if "something goes wrong." So, childbirth it is. I must be conscious. I must go through three stages: dilation of the cervix, contractions, and expulsion of the fetus.

On the preggy-weggy sites, they write that the pain of labor is nothing compared to the happiness you experience at finally seeing your "little one."

I won't see my little one. I don't want to see him. I don't want that ugly, deformed, innocent, murdered being to appear to me later in endless nightmares. I warn everyone—Natasha, my husband, the midwives, the doctors—I do not want, I do not want to look at him, not for anything. When it's all over, please, let him be taken away immediately, and I'll close my eyes. Natasha, translate this for them, please. In case they suddenly don't understand English.

They understand. They say: okay, everything will happen the way you say. But it's not right. You should look at him.

"I don't want to, I'm afraid to look at him," I say to Sasha. "That's the worst thing of all! Promise me I won't have to do that!"

"I promise. No one's planning to force you to do it."

"And you aren't afraid to see him?!"

"No, An. I'm not afraid. I'm afraid of other things entirely."

"What things?"

"Complications. Hemorrhages. You know what things..."

For some reason, I'm not much afraid of complications. I'm afraid to see him. And I'm also afraid of the shot that will kill him.

Twelve-thirty. We sit in the room—I, my husband, Natasha. Half an hour ago, they began inducing labor. The method of inducing is very gentle—one tablet of misoprostol administered vaginally every three hours. The midwife administers it quickly and painlessly right there in the room, I don't even have to sit in the gynecological chair.

"We hope this will be sufficient and that your contractions will start somewhere after the third or fourth tablet."

"And if they don't start?"

"There are other methods of inducing labor. But women generally respond well to this drug."

"And when will the shot be... the poison shot?"

"You're very frightened of that shot?"

"Yes."

"I'll ask the doctor."

I "respond" even better than they expect. Light contractions begin after the first tablet. After the second—at three p.m.—they become regular. They offer me an epidural, but the pain's bearable, and I refuse. They say that if it's easier for me, they'll cancel the lethal shot. They've compared the anticipated weight of the fetus and the intensity of the contractions and concluded that the baby will die pretty quickly on his own.

With relief, I agree. I don't ask how difficult death will be. I'll allow him to "die on his own"—as if in the natural course of things, as if I took no part in it – and to this day, I can't forgive myself for it. What I've just done doesn't immediately occur to me. It's much later. When we finally receive the autopsy report (at Charité, this takes a long time) and Natasha, having first stopped short, translates the cause of death for me: "a massive hemorrhage in the brain."

... After the third tablet, at six p.m., serious pain begins. On the nightstand next to my bed sit the stuffed dog and the meerkat, the talismans my daughter gave me to bring with me, but they don't help. I agree to the epidural and, in a couple of minutes, cold-eyed Kai comes into the room. They attach me to equipment that records my blood pressure and pulse (with an epidural during ordinary labor, they also follow the fetal heartbeat, but in our case, no one worries about that), Kai prepares my back with something icy. Now, he needs to place the needle in my spine with precision, for that I need to sit still, without moving. But I can't sit still. I writhe from the contractions and tremble heavily from fear. Not Sasha's exhortations, not his stroking, not regular breathing, not a sedative, not Kai's assurances that I'll just feel a light "bzzz—like a mosquito bite," nothing helps. Then, the indifferent Kai manages an astonishing feat:

"I was in Moscow as a child," he says to me in English. "I remember Moscow as having a large number of monuments. Ever since then, the question has bothered me: how many are there? Can you tell me even approximately the number of monuments in Moscow?"

Introducing the unexpected is, in my case, an excellent method of distraction. While I'm vaguely astonished to myself at his heartlessness (what the hell is wrong with him, monuments at such a terrible moment?), while I nevertheless politely try to come up with a figure and consider what this person understands by the term "monument," he's able to stick the needle where it needs to go. And he immediately loses all interest in the monuments of Russia's capital. But the pain goes away. Quickly, and almost completely.

I continue to feel contractions—but already, this isn't pain, just the shadow of pain. My legs feel slightly numb, as if I've been sitting on them too long. Kai says I can walk around if I want to, but only with support. But best of all would be to sit or lie down.

"Find something to occupy yourself with," he advises. "Do you have a computer with you? Excellent. Watch a movie."

Again, I'm astounded by his heartlessness. When Kai leaves, the midwife checks my blood pressure and also leaves. Sasha falls asleep—it's instantly, and without warning, as if he's been unplugged from a socket (I've always been amazed by his ability to turn off in stressful situations), and Natasha and I sit silently for a little while and stare at my I.V., and then she says:

"Maybe we really should try to watch something?"

There's no internet at Charité, it's not possible to download or watch online. It turns out that the only film in my laptop is *The Three Musketeers* with Mikhail Boyarsky, at some time I downloaded it for my daughter.

And so, Natasha and I sit on the couch in the German Charité clinic, me with an I.V., I'm giving birth to a baby who'll never take a breath, his father sleeps like the dead next to me, and we watch *The Three Musketeers*, where they fence, fall in love, and drink. It turns out later that from that day forward and forever after, *The Three Musketeers* becomes the most frightening film I've ever seen in my life, I'll never watch it again. And the ditty about *It's time, it's time to rejoice in life* and *Bye-bye, bye-bye, feathers waving high* is the most terrifying song in the world, and I can't bear to hear it ever again. I'll turn off the sound if it's played on the Children's Radio channel, I'll leave the room if someone sings it. For me, it's a song about how unborn children die, and with them dies all the happiness in the world; for me, it's a song about how fate spits on your wishes; for me, it's a song about how my little son says *Bye-bye* to me...

But all that comes later. Now, I simply stare at the screen and almost nod off and even almost forget why I'm here. And then—all of a sudden, in an instant—I remember. Because through the drowsiness, through the hat feathers waving high, through the painkillers, through my numb stomach, I suddenly feel that something inside me is tearing away and ceasing to live. Inside me is—death. It's hot, slippery, red, it moves rhythmically inside me as if dancing, it wants to tear me open and come out.

"The baby's coming," I say to Natasha and push the call button for the midwife.

Everything after that takes place as if in the theater. As if we've already rehearsed the scene more than once. The midwife instantly appears in the room with a tray and a baby blanket. Sasha wakes up, immediately leaps up, and stands on the other side of the bed, behind me, and strokes my face. And Natasha steps a little off to the side and looks at us. She doesn't have children yet, and I don't want her to see this kind of birth. I'm able to ask her to turn away, and she turns, and I feel how death flows down my legs, and then, I begin to scream. Not from pain. From fear.

Through my own screams, I hear how the midwife is speaking German and Natasha, standing with her back to me, translates very calmly and quietly. She says it's almost over. Very soon, it will be all over. But for that to happen, I have to stop screaming. I have to exhale, then inhale, exhale again, and push. But I don't have to scream. I don't have to scream.

I listen to Natasha's voice, I exhale, inhale. Death is born with the first push, in silence. And my baby comes with it. I don't scream—and he doesn't scream. My eyes are closed—and his probably are, too.

"Everything came out, even the placenta," says the midwife, and I somehow understand her before Natasha translates. "Do you want to see the baby?"

"No, I don't."

I feel how the midwife quickly and deftly catches and wraps the baby blanket around something slippery, moist, cooling that lies between my legs—death, the placenta, and the dead baby boy—everything that's come out of me. And she also deftly pulls waterproof underwear onto me.

"This isn't right," says the midwife, and again I understand without the translation. "I've worked here for twenty years. I've seen many women like you. Those women who refuse to look at the baby later lose their peace of mind forever. They come back here after a few months or years, they make inquiries and cry, they want to see their children, but it's too late then."

"I don't want to look at him."

"As you wish. You can open your eyes now."

I open my eyes, and she leaves with the tray and a bundle.

"Did you see him?" I ask Sasha.

"No, they took him away... so quickly."

"Where did they take him?"

"I don't know," says Sasha.

"Do you know where they took him, Natasha?"

She doesn't know.

I become terrified. Because they took him away all wrapped up, took him along the hospital corridors to a cold, unknown place.

The midwife returns without the bundle, she says something to me, but I no longer understand German.

"Now, they'll do an ultrasound," Natasha translates. "They want to be certain nothing remains in your uterus."

I try to stand up, but the midwife gestures to me to lie back down, on my back, with my arms crossed on my chest. I don't like this pose, it's the pose dead people assume, I put my hands behind my head, but the midwife comes up and returns them to their former position. They wheel the ultrasound into the room on a cart, someone runs the sensor across my stomach to clarify whether anything remains in my uterus and whether I need "some surgery," but I'm not worried about that. My main concern is not to lie in this pose, like a corpse. I put my hands behind my head again and again, and again and again the midwife crosses them on my chest and speaks in a foreign language.

"She asks you to hold your arms this way," says Natasha. "It's better for your blood circulation."

I give up and hold still in the pose of a corpse. They're right – it's the most becoming pose for me. Death was inside me and, probably, it didn't all come out. Something of it remained. Some fragments and clots.

"There's nothing in the uterus," says the ultrasound doctor. "You're fortunate. You won't need any surgery."

She wipes the gel from my stomach, where my baby no longer is, where nothing is any longer, except the traces death left behind. Those traces can't be seen on the ultrasound, but I feel them. I really feel them in myself.

They leave—both the midwife and the ultrasound doctor—and I lie with crossed arms and look at the ceiling. Natasha also says goodbye and leaves—it's already late at night.

My Sasha leans over me and asks:

"How are you doing?"

"I think I'm dying," I say to my Sasha. "He died—and I'm dying now, too. Can that be?"

"No, it can't," says Sasha. "The doctors would have noticed if you were dying."

"It feels as if there's no air in here," I say. "It's hard to breathe. I'm cold. My lips are growing numb. And my nose. And my cheeks."

"Should I call the doctor?"

"Call the doctor."

My Sasha leaves—and comes back with Kai, the lover of monuments. Kai has a syringe in his hand filled with clear liquid, he glances at the sensor that's still measuring my blood pressure and pulse, and says:

"Physically, you're fine. But you're experiencing stress. If you don't object, I'll give you something to calm you."

"I don't object."

About five minutes after the shot, air returns to the room, and the feeling returns to me that my face is my face and not a death mask. After about another ten minutes comes the understanding that the baby and I are no longer one. I'm alive—and he's dead. It's he and not I who doesn't breathe and doesn't feel his own skin...

It's he who lies alone now in the cold, with his face covered up. No one knows him. No one needs him. No one has hugged him.

"Maybe we should have looked at him, no matter what?" I say to Sasha.

"Maybe."

"But I'm afraid that he's very scary. That I'll dream about him the rest of my life."

"Let's do this," says Sasha. "I'll go by myself now, find out where he is, and I'll look at him. And then, I'll tell you whether he's scary or not. And whether you can look at him."

I feel much easier that Sasha will now find him, be with him, and look in his face. And also, that when he comes back, he'll say whether or not I can look at my dead son without losing my mind. I'm certain my husband will determine this correctly.

My husband comes back with red eyes and says:

"He's not scary."

"What, not scary at all?"

"Not at all. But he's... sad. And I'm very sorry for him. Look at him."

Chapter 13
Seeing the Baby

At seven in the morning, a nurse with the eyes of a fawn wakes me.

"Breakfast time." She places a tray of breakfast on the small table next to my bed.

I surface from a dream that's heavy and black as a tombstone, and in the first seconds, I can't figure out where I am or what's happened to me. Sasha is sleeping in the neighboring bed, snoring. The nurse-fawn smiles so radiantly that it feels as if something wonderful has happened.

"Do you want to see your baby?" she asks.

Well, of course, I want to see my... I even manage to smile at her before I remember: last night I gave birth to a dead baby. At whom I didn't look.

"Do you want to see your little baby?" she repeats.

"Yes. I do," I answer hoarsely, and together with the words, blood gushes out, a lot of blood. "When?"

"After breakfast."

"I don't want anything to eat."

"How can that be—you don't want to eat?" The fawn opens her eyes wide in amazement. "It's breakfast. You have to eat at least something. And you also have to take this pill. So you don't start lactating."

Sasha wakes up. I cram toast with butter and jam into myself, coffee with milk, and the pill—so I won't produce any milk. The nurse-fawn returns and invites us to follow her. And she smiles anew, in such a way that it's as if they're waiting for us at a school play. I follow her, and blood flows out of me, warm and thick, like humus. Last night, it was still our shared blood—mine and my son's. Today, it's just my blood, and for me alone, it's too much. Today, I'm going to look at him. At my son. At my little baby.

I'm certain that we're going to the morgue, but Fawn leads us into a comfortable room with a sofa, coffee table, and a picture on the wall and asks us to wait just a minute. She leaves—and in a couple of minutes, she returns with a wicker basket decorated with artificial flowers. She places the basket on the coffee table, right in front of me.

There in the basket, surrounded by plastic flowers, covered in a light blue blanket, lies a little baby in a cap. He looks like Sasha. He has a sad and hurt face.

Tightly closed eyes. Barely noticeable, knitted brows. Tiny lips, pursed as if to cry out, a cry that will never be uttered. A cry that I must not, cannot hear—but all the same, I hear it. I look at his unmoving face and calmly, without fear, am amazed that I hear a dead child whimpering, thinly and quietly, but absolutely clearly.

"Of course, cry, if that makes it easier," says the nurse-fawn, and it suddenly dawns on me that *I* am making those sounds. It's me whimpering, not the dead baby in the basket.

"You can touch him," she says. "You can hold him in your arms. Don't be afraid. It's not frightening at all. Like this."

She takes my dead baby out of the basket and lays him across my knees. I touch his face lightly. It's cold. It's very cold. I stroke that cold face and howl. To the touch, his forehead feels like pastry dough that's spent the night in the refrigerator.

"He looks like you," I say to Sasha, "our baby."

"It seems so, yes. Did I do the right thing in telling you to look at him?"

"You did everything right."

We sit and look at our dead son. Between us is—trust. The maximum trust and closeness that's possible between people. Somewhere, in another life, another world, is that stubborn, alien, frightened man who tried to convince me that "it's just an embryo" and "an unfortunate pregnancy, like an ectopic one," and hoped to soothe me with that. This one, mine, is real, honest, and brave—he was with me all the way.

There are no precise statistics, but a great number of marriages in Russia collapse after the late termination of a pregnancy. And I know why. Because husbands remain forever at the "just an embryo" and "unfortunate pregnancy" stage. Because they don't let husbands into gynecological clinics. Or into hospitals. Or let them be present at birth. Or let them look at the baby. At the dead baby. Not at an embryo.

Administrators don't let them in because they have instructions dating back to the Inquisition, and it's plainly written there that in that grief, a husband and wife mustn't be together, but separate. Furthermore, that grief for some reason mustn't be called grief, but exclusively a "fetal pathology."

Doctors and nurses don't let them in because they also have instructions, and they don't give a damn about the abyss that inevitably gapes open between a man who stubbornly talks about "just an embryo" and a woman who gives birth, in torment, to a dead baby with a little mouth shaped in an expression of suffering.

Even women themselves don't let them in because their mothers, grandmothers, great-grandmothers have told them that this is God's punishment. And that it's shameful to look at such a thing or talk about such a thing. That a "real man," seeing "such a thing" (or even hearing about "such a thing"), will immediately run away. They don't let them in, they suffer, they're silent, hoping to buy God's forgiveness with that silence and hold onto that "real man." But it's wrong, it's impossible to be together when "such a thing" is between you. Such grief. Such an abyss. When you're on opposite sides of it.

CHAPTER 14
IN LOVING MEMORY

They discharge me from the clinic that same day.

Before discharge, Sasha and I give blood samples that have to be forwarded from Charité to the Institute of Human Genetics in Aachen to search for a mutation in the PKHD1 gene. They'll be looking at the "hot spots"—that is, analyzing those sections of the gene in which the genetic mutation responsible for the development of infantile polycystic kidney disease most often occurs. If we "get lucky" and they find the mutation in both me and Sasha, during our next pregnancy, we can undergo genetic testing. And if the embryo again inherits the damage from both of us, we can abort before the twelfth week. Moreover, it's even possible to do in vitro fertilization. The cells are fertilized outside the uterus, the embryos are again checked, and only healthy ones are implanted.

If they don't find any damage, our risk of a repeat occurrence will always be 25 percent. It's very simple—like the problem of predicting brown-eyed and blue-eyed children taught in school. For example, you have a brown-eyed mama and a brown-eyed papa: the gene for brown eyes is dominant, it will be expressed. But we know that each of them has a blue-eyed parent who passed them the recessive (that is, passive, not outwardly expressed) gene for blue eyes. What's the probability that these two brown-eyed people will give birth to a blue-eyed boy? If the dominant brown eyes of the mama combine with the dominant brown eyes of the papa, the boy's eyes will be brown. If the dominant brown eyes of one parent combine with the recessive blue eyes of the other, the child's eyes will be brown anyway, as the dominant gene controls. But if the two recessive genes for blue eyes combine, the boy will turn out to have blue eyes. The probability of this, therefore, is one in four.

I don't know what color eyes our son has. What color eyes our son had. Grey, probably. Because Sasha and I and our daughter have grey eyes. However, each of us probably has the recessive gene for blue eyes. Just like the recessive gene for polycystic kidney disease. And if my recessive (that is, not expressed) gene for polycystic kidney disease combines with Sasha's recessive gene for polycystic kidney disease, the result will be a dead boy. Another dead boy with enormous kidneys. And the likelihood of that is one in four.

"Well, good luck," the attending doctor shakes our hands. "I very much hope to see you again in our clinic, but on a more joyous occasion. If you get pregnant, come to us again. We'll send the autopsy results by mail. We'll also inform you of the date and place of your baby's burial. You can come to the funeral, if you like."

"And...you'll prescribe antibiotics for me?"

"Why? You don't have an infection."

"But... in Russia they always prescribe a course of antibiotics in these cases. As a precaution."

"We don't do that. Why upset the workings of the body for no reason?"

"And... I'll have to come back in a few days for an exam?"

"Only if something unexpected happens. Otherwise, a regular checkup in a month or two. You'll most likely be in Moscow. And this is for you." She holds out a sealed envelope to me.

"What's inside?"

"A little something to remember your baby by."

I pull my hand back from the envelope.

"Don't be afraid. There's nothing scary inside. Just a photo. We have evidence that women feel much better when they have the ability to look at a photo of their baby sometimes."

I take the envelope—but I don't open it that day, or the day after.

On the third day, I'm drinking coffee with cream in our Berlin rental apartment—and suddenly, I experience such a strong tidal wave of sorrow that my chest hurts, and my shirt becomes wet around my nipples. My sorrow is that white, warm milk that there's no one to drink.

For some reason, my sorrow isn't treated by the hormone pill that suppresses lactation.

I go into the bathroom, stand under the shower, and express the milk. Milk and blood pour out of me. The water in the bottom of the tub turns brown.

And then, I return and unseal the envelope in which there's something "to remember my baby by." I look at his face. At his hurt, pursed lips that will never touch my breast. Besides the photo, there's also some kind of paper in the envelope, folded in two. I open it up—and see the ink print of a tiny hand and a tiny foot.

They smeared blue ink on my son's palm, cold like yesterday's dough, and pressed it to this paper.

I touch this paper with my lips. This inky palm. A new helping of sorrow spreads two wet spots over my shirt.

The next day, I'll take one more pill for suppressing lactation. After that, the milk will disappear. But not the sorrow.

CHAPTER 15
PANIC

I feel fine, nothing hurts, I don't have a temperature, and with each passing day, there's less blood. After about ten days, we buy tickets to Moscow. We stand in line at the check-in counter. The closer we get to the Aeroflot counter, the harder something tugs inside me. As if the thinnest, invisible piece of elastic connects me to German soil. A piece of elastic stretching between my solar plexus and my baby, who'll be buried in this soil. I thought all my connections with him had been broken—but no, this connection still remained and is just now breaking. The connection is purely geographic. He's remaining here—and I'm flying away.

We check in for the flight, go through the metal detector—and the invisible elastic snaps. It's painful. Like it always is when elastic that's stretched tight breaks.

The first panic attack—however, I don't yet know that's what it is—happens to me here, in the airport, in the line for passport control. The oxygen suddenly disappears. I breathe, I inhale something, but it's not air, it's emptiness. There is no air. And my heart pounds in my ears. I tell Sasha I'm suffocating. That I can't breathe at all. He looks attentively at me and says:

"No, you're breathing."

He opens a flask of whisky bought in the duty-free shop.

"Drink. Take three big swallows."

I obediently take three swallows, he stows the whisky away, and he hugs me. I hide my nose and mouth in his sweater—and somehow, it's easier to breathe in that position. As if, instead of too little air, there'd been too much—and now there's just enough.

Chapter 16
Conspiracy of Silence

... We're traveling somewhere on a train—my two children and I. I have a girl and a boy. With the girl, everything's clear—it's Sasha Little Badger. But the son makes me a little anxious. He's probably around two years old, but I can't say, exactly. No matter how hard I try, I can't see his face. His back is to me all the time: he turns away, laughing. He runs away from me on the train car, stomping his bare feet amusingly. He presses his nose to the window, and I see only the downy back of his head. And then somehow, entirely without my participation, all at once, my children are suddenly sound asleep. My daughter's in the upper berth, uncovered, as always. I pull the covers over her and kiss her forehead. My son's in the lower berth. He lies on his stomach, having buried his face in the pillow. I squat down next to him, smooth his hair, hoping he'll turn his head towards me—but he's motionless. I think about whether to turn him on his back so I can finally find out how he looks. I don't want to wake him—but on the other hand, it really isn't normal that I have no idea what the child's face looks like. What color are his eyes, for example? How can it be that I haven't once in my life looked into his eyes? Does that kind of thing even happen? And by the way, where are we going on this train? What's my son's name? I'm frightened that I don't remember such simple things. I strain every nerve trying to remember—and with that strain, both boy and train disappear. And I wake up.

... Every night, I dream sorrowful, anxious dreams.

In these dreams, I'm wandering around various strange apartments, corridors, basements, and vestibules and painfully trying to remember what I've forgotten there. Something important. Phone? Purse? Textbook? Keys? The dog? None of those. It seems I've lost something else...

In these dreams, I'm running around some kind of beautiful street, it's pleasant that I'm running quickly, lightly. And then, I'm suddenly astonished: where does this lightness come from? Am I not pregnant? Where's my enormous, heavy stomach?...

In these dreams, I choose toys in a children's store—but no matter how hard I try, I can't recollect to whom I'm planning to give them. Toy airplanes and cars—probably to some little boy...

In these dreams, I see a boy from behind—and don't remember what color his eyes are...

And then, I remember—and wake up.

... Moscow. February 2013. I have only a daughter. There's no large, heavy stomach. There's no happy son pressing his nose to the window and stomping his bare feet. There might have been—but there isn't. It's a son—and not my keys or the dog—that I've lost. What should have been my son was born two months ago, was never named, lay a month in a German morgue awaiting autopsy, was cut open, sewn up again, and was recently buried in a common grave in a Berlin cemetery with other children born dead. I don't know the exact date of the funeral, don't know where the cemetery is, how the grave looks, what kind of people were at the burial and whether they brought toys to the grave. Toy airplanes and cars. In Berlin, Natasha has a letter about the funeral from the Charité clinic. She asked whether to open it or not—I said there was no need.

She also received a letter with the autopsy report—that one, I asked her to read to me. In that letter, it said the fetus—of the male sex, weighing three hundred and sixty grams—had bilateral diffuse multicystic dysplastic kidney. And resulting underdevelopment of the ureter, bladder, and lungs. And in the letter, it said the cause of death was a hemorrhage of the brain. Nothing was said in the letter about the color of his eyes. That means I'll never know. But I think they're grey. Like ours.

Like ours and our daughter's.

In spite of what the psychologist said, our daughter for some reason doesn't ask us any questions. None. As if nothing had happened. As if we'd simply had a Christmas holiday, and Papa and I went to visit the Christmas markets in Berlin, and she went to stay with her grandmother and grandfather. As if there hadn't been any pregnancy, no little brother whom she planned to call Littlest Badger, no stuffed talismans tucked into my suitcase "to help"... I wait a little while for questions—and then I myself ask:

"Maybe you want to talk about what happened?"

"What, did something happen to someone?" An open felt-tip marker twirls in her hand.

"Well, yes. Happened. To us. To our baby."

She's silent. She pulls at the marker. Her palms and fingers are covered in red spots.

I make another attempt.

"Maybe you want to ask me something?"

"No, I don't want to. Or, well, I want to. But I can't."

"Why?"

"Grandma and Grandfather told me very strictly not to talk to you about... not to talk about... the baby. And not to ask you about anything ever, not for any reason."

"Why?!"

"They said I mustn't remind you about it. So you can forget about it more quickly."

I smile. This is so wild, it's practically funny. "Not remind you about it." Seriously? What am I, senile? What does "not remind you" mean when it's the only thing I can think about? Nonetheless, not just my parents, but just about everyone with whom I interact holds to this remarkable principle of "not reminding me." People who until our trip searched for doctors, called and wrote every day, asked how I felt and what the ultrasound showed—these same people surround me with a solid circle of silence when I return from Berlin to Moscow.

That is, no, they aren't formally silent. They talk to me about the weather, about movies, about how Sasha's doing in school. They all put up the same pretense— and obviously want me to pretend the same thing—that nothing's happened. They assiduously avoid themes of childbirth and, especially, babies born dead. And if I myself try to tell them something about what happened, they're frightened, they fidget, avert their eyes, they suddenly have to make an important phone call and, by the way, is it true that my book was translated into Spanish and has done well in Spain? They consider it their duty to "distract" me.

I don't want to be distracted. I don't want to "forget about it more quickly." I want to remember. I want to talk about my dead baby. All conversations on extraneous subjects seem pointless to me. It doesn't make things better for me when they distract me, it makes things harder. Sometimes, I correspond with or talk on the phone to Natasha—but it's not the same, she's too far away. I talk with my husband—but he's in the middle of the situation, and that's not the same, either. Only once did a friend who'd just given birth (just a few months ago, both of us pregnant, we discussed how our little boys would be friends—our older daughters are already friends)—only once did she visit me and start asking me how everything went at Charité. How I gave birth. And how I felt. And who he turned out to look like.

She listened to me for three hours. I talked, and it made things better for me. But she has a nursing son, she has the milk, it's time to feed him. She left—and the circle of silence and forgetting closed around me again.

... Still, I pulled my daughter from that circle. I told her I was prepared for any question. That it would even be a joy to speak with her about it, if she wanted to. That I needed and wanted to remember, because our Littlest Badger was worthy of having us remember him.

And then she asks:

"Mama, did it hurt?"

And I tell her, no. Physically, it didn't really hurt at all. But it hurt my soul.

"And did it hurt him? My little brother?"

And I tell her, yes. Probably, yes. Because they anesthetized me, and not him.

She cries. And then, she asks if the same thing will happen to her when she wants to have a baby.

I tell her it's unlikely. I tell her about chance, probability, and risk. I explain to her, as best I can, about genetic mutations. I tell her that even if she's a carrier of the gene with the mutation, the chance that her husband will also have the mutation is exceedingly low.

I tell her that soon we'll receive the results of the blood test. And if the geneticists find our mutation, then they'll be able to test her for it, they'll know exactly where and what to look for. And to some degree, that will protect her in the future. To some degree, that will also protect us the next time we try to have a baby.

"And you're going to try?" Her eyes open wide with amazement and happiness. "You are going to try, right?"

CHAPTER 17
FIFTY–FIFTY

The tests for mutations come back "empty": the geneticists didn't find anything in me or my husband. "This doesn't mean that you don't have mutations," it says in the accompanying letter. "It means that we didn't find them in the most probable locations where they're most often encountered with polycystic kidney disease. Your chances for a repeat occurrence: 25 percent."

After a couple of days, another letter arrives from them, by email. It says they received the autopsy report, in which "multicystic dysplastic kidney" and not "polycystic kidney disease" is specified, and that changes things. A different gene is responsible for multicystic dysplastic kidney. They promise to carry out a new test.

We wait another month. New results come back—and again, they show nothing. They didn't find anything. This doesn't mean that we don't have mutations, it says in the accompanying letter. It means that they didn't find mutations in the most probable locations. If it's multicystic dysplastic kidney, then dominant inheritance is not ruled out. In that case, the probability of a repeat occurrence is up to 50 percent. Up to 50 percent. Multicystic dysplastic kidney has different forms, often milder ones, often only on one side, and then the prognosis for life is favorable. But as a rule, if birth defects recur, they're often just as serious as the first time.

"Up to 50 percent," I say to my husband, in English. "Look at the chance we now have for a repeat occurrence."

"I don't want a repeat occurrence," says Sasha, gloomily. "Maybe we don't need a second baby so badly? We already have one child. If you want, we can get a dog. You've always wanted a dog. Maybe Little Badger and a dog are enough?"

"Not enough for me," I say. "I really need that baby. I'll never be happy if I don't give birth to a live baby."

"But, Anya. A 50 percent chance that nightmare will happen again. That's a lot. That's really a lot!"

"A 50 percent chance I'll give birth and everything will be normal," I say, stubbornly. "That's also a lot."

"I can't imagine how we'll go on living if all that happens again."

"And I can't imagine how I'll go on living if I don't have a baby."

"I don't know. I'm not ready."

"But... we already agreed! We really wanted to try."

"We wanted to wait for the test results—and try after that."

"Well, we waited for the results!"

"These aren't the results we were waiting for!"

... We acquire a puppy. A funny red poodle. We call him Kokos. I teach him various commands. He licks my hands. He walks on his hind legs. Little Badger and Kokos play well together. But it isn't enough for me.

"Please, let's try anyway," I say to Sasha every day.

"I don't know," Sasha turns gloomy. "I've got to think about it."

I walk with the happy puppy along the banks of the Moscow River and look attentively at the brown ice breaking in the black water, so as not to look at the women with baby carriages. They all, all have baby carriages. Or giant stomachs.

CHAPTER 18
SPACE WITHOUT AIR

The end of April. The puppy has grown noticeably. I don't talk about pregnancy any more. I really want a baby, it's my *idée fixe*, but it's laughable to even think about pregnancy now. Not because Sasha's against it—on the whole, I've talked him around—but because of me. My body's against it. I've turned out to be the weak link, not Sasha.

I break down, I'm constantly sick. Something's not right with my body. It's possible that I've got something incurable, terrible. Something fatal. Probably something stayed inside me that night at Charité when I gave birth to a dead fetus of the male sex weighing three hundred and sixty grams. Some kind of tiny, unnoticed, microscopic offshoot of death remained inside then, in place of the fetus—and all these months it's been growing, growing, developing, and now it's killing me. The closer May comes—I was supposed to give birth to my son in May— the worse I get.

It's hard for me to breathe. At first, I experience attacks of breathlessness once every few days; then, every day; then, three, four, five, eight times a day. It's hard for me to swallow. I'm practically unable to eat, I lose weight. I eat yogurt and cheese once a day. No other food will go down—not in the figurative, but in the most literal sense: I simply can't swallow it. I can't sleep. I can't climb the stairs to the fourth floor. My pulse beats furiously. My head spins, my eyes go dark, my hands go numb, and my blood pressure races.

I drink whisky, valerian, Anaprilin, and tranquilizers—sometimes separately, sometimes together. I check my pulse and blood pressure. I go to doctors. An endless medical "bad trip": MRI, gastroscopy, blood tests, ultrasound, x-rays. I take Little Sasha to doctors: she complains it's hard for her to breathe, too. Her head hurts, and she feels nauseous. I'm afraid she's also got something bad. I read about my own and her symptoms on the web—and I see these are the symptoms of terrible illnesses.

But they don't find anything—nothing that could exhibit these symptoms. But the symptoms don't disappear. And if they remain at approximately the same level for Little Badger—not affecting her attendance at school, on long walks, or on visits— then I just get worse every day. I practically don't get out anywhere. I walk the dog not far from our building's entryway, and generally don't walk at all. I'm afraid to leave home alone because I'll start gasping for air, and no one will be able to help me. I'm afraid to visit people because I'll start gasping in front of everyone, and they'll all look at me. I'm afraid to go to a café because I won't be able to swallow my salad. I refuse to give readings—there are too many strangers, outsiders, my blood pressure will race, and my pulse will go off the charts. I practically don't see people. Big Sasha fusses over me like a good nanny. And over Little Badger. And over the dog.

Sometimes I try to "get hold of myself," overcome my fears, and complete some kind of feat. For example, to walk to the Dove Café, it's ten minutes from home, and buy some fresh-baked pizza there. Especially because a friend has at long last promised to drop in this evening. Before going out, I drink three sips of whisky—for ten minutes, the whisky relaxes me. I don't risk going anywhere without three sips of whisky. I walk along the street, trying to stand up straight and breathe evenly. I tell myself everything's fine with my lungs, that's what the doctors said. I tell myself it's nice on the street. It's spring on the street. Birds sing on the street. Buds are opening up, sticky, furled leaflets are showing themselves—like babies from the womb. My baby should have been born in a couple of weeks. And should have seen these sticky leaflets and breathed in this air. But, no. He wouldn't have been able to breathe. His lungs wouldn't open up... I try to imagine how lungs open up. How they actually breathe. How they contract... I try to breathe evenly, but the air stops. I look around me. I'm in the exact middle of the path between home and the pizza. From inside, panic hits me in a hot, noisy wave, knocks me off my feet, catches me and tosses me into the deep. I sit on a bench. Blood pulses in my head. I touch my cheeks, my nose—and I don't feel my skin. I check my pulse—it's one hundred and thirty. I want to phone Sasha, ask him to come get me and take me home—but I restrain myself. What the hell's wrong with me? Am I really not able to buy pizza? I pull an Anaprilin from my handbag and place it beneath my tongue. Anaprilin is extremely bitter. So bitter that it distracts even me. I suck on the pill and wait while my heart begins to beat more slowly. I sit on that bench for about forty minutes, maybe an hour. Then the attack passes, I go to the Dove Café, order the pizza, wait twenty minutes, take the box, and head home. At the halfway point from the Dove Café to home, it all happens again. I sit on the bench. Devour Anaprilin. Gasp for air.

It's already dark when I arrive home with the cold, stiff pizza. My husband and the guest are on the balcony, smoking and drinking dry red wine. I hand them the pizza; my hands shake. Sasha warms the pizza in the oven, we sit down at the table. They eat—and I don't. I can't swallow that pizza. Our friend Andrey looks at me attentively—and asks if everything's all right.

"Aside from the fact that I can't breathe, eat, or sleep, everything's all right."

With great interest, he asks questions to clarify things and find out details. He's a writer like we are—and I languidly consider what's awakened his interest.

Maybe some kind of minor character in his unfinished book is withering away, and as a writer he's just lacking some texture for the character.

"You have neurosis," he concludes, contentedly. "You need a psychologist. I also had neurosis. I know what I'm talking about."

Chapter 19
It Didn't Worry Me at All

The psychologist is named Angelina. She has excellent recommendations. She sees patients in her own office near the Belorusskaya metro station. Her schedule's packed. She's in demand. She's expensive.

Our first session goes a little strangely. She wonders what brought me to her, and I tell her about the pregnancy termination; about my current problems with breathing, sleeping, and eating; about the fruitless parade of doctor visits.

She listens, nods, then makes a wise face and says, with the intonation of Sherlock Holmes, speaking frankly for the first time with the slow-witted Watson:

"This is all about death. You're talking about death, Anna!"

It seems she's waiting for me to applaud.

"Well, of course, it's all about death," I agree, bored. "I really am talking to you about death."

Angelina looks disappointed. But she doesn't back down:

"You're afraid of death, Anna. Isn't that so?"

"Well, yes. I've been telling you that for nearly thirty minutes already."

"And you experience anxiety.

"Yes! I experience anxiety!"

She nods sagely.

"Well, Anna. Let's think about what kind of help you want from me."

"I want professional psychological help from you."

"So, try to express what kind of expectations you have. What kind of result do you want to achieve?"

"I want to achieve the result of not suffocating and not experiencing problems with eating and sleeping."

She smiles, craftily:

"In psychology, we think negative formulations shouldn't be used in speech. And here you say: 'I want to achieve *not...*'"

"Fine. I want to achieve normal breathing, normal eating, and sound sleeping. Does that work?"

Angelina nods wisely and goes quiet. I get the unpleasant suspicion that she doesn't fully understand what to do with me and really does expect some kind of plan from me. I'm silent. Sighing, she takes the initiative into her own hands.

"In your situation, it makes sense to take antidepressants. In connection, of course, with psychotherapy sessions."

"I don't want to take antidepressants."

"Why?"

"Because as far as I know, antidepressants are taken over a long period of time, around a year. And I mustn't get pregnant while taking them."

"So, you want to get pregnant? After that?!" She looks at me as if I'm a psychopath. Which, by the way, is probably the case. She's the psychotherapist, and I'm the psychopath, we've found one another in an office near the Belorusskaya metro station.

"Yes, I do."

"Well... Then, we'll try to work without antidepressants."

"Excellent."

"That's all for today. You absolutely must fill out these forms before the next session. Among other things, there's a scale for measuring anxiety and depression. It's a very important part of our work, please take the form seriously."

The form I try to fill out at home is capable of plunging anyone—even the happiest, most successful, and flourishing person, surrounded by a throng of loving children and grandchildren—into anxiety and depression. It's an endless series of boring and stupid questions translated by Google Translate or God-knows-what from God-knows-which language, and for the most part, it bears absolutely no relation to me personally.

"I'm glad today same as before." The answers range from:
1. Yes, of course.
2. Yes, but not as much.
3. It worried me a bit.
4. It didn't worry me at all.

"I feel myself happy."
Yes, of course.
Yes, but not as much.
It worried me a bit.
It didn't worry me at all.

"I can simply sit down, and relaxed."
Yes, of course.
Yes, but not as much.

It worried me a bit.

It didn't worry me at all.

Swearing quietly under my breath, I check "It didn't worry me at all."

On the next form, the questions are more complicated. There, you don't just have to put checks, but also write answers to the questions.

"In the near future, I want to be..." Write what you want to be. For example: "I want to be slim/trim/happy/self-confident/successful in my career." Try to avoid negative formulations. You shouldn't write "I don't want to be so fat/have my belly hanging out, etc."

At that, I break down. At the next session, I tell Angelina I don't see the sense of answering questions addressed to the collective woman of forty-plus who feels inadequate because of idleness or extra weight.

Angelina is slightly offended on behalf of her clients.

"By the way, according to this form that you *did* fill out, it's clear you have a very high level of anxiety."

"I don't doubt it. That's clear, even without the form."

"If you like, I'll show you several relaxation techniques used to treat anxiety disorders. They'll help you reduce stress. And regulate your breathing."

"Yes, I'd like that very much!" I think, with relief, that possibly something useful will come from Angelina.

She asks me to lie on my back, close my eyes, lay my arms on my chest, and lie still. Without moving. To sink completely into myself, renouncing the external world.

...I lie on my back, with my arms crossed on my chest. As I did then, at Charité, immediately after giving birth. I lie in that same pose again, like a corpse. Probably, it's the most suitable pose for me...

"And now, hold your breath."

... I lie with my arms crossed—I don't move and don't breathe. Suddenly, it seems to me that I'll never breathe again. Even if I want to. Even if Angelina says I can.

I leap up and gasp for air.

"What happened?" Angelina's frightened.

"I can't do this! I can't lie on my back and hold my breath."

... We politely say goodbye until next week. We both know that I won't be coming back.

CHAPTER 20
THE WICKED WITCH AND THE BABY WITHOUT A NAME

On the other hand, I find a really good child psychologist for Little Badger. Natalya Kurenkova works in the Yugo-Zapadny Center for Psychological, Medical, and Social Support. Little Badger and I finally arrive at her office on the third attempt: the first two end in fiasco because the closer we get to the metro, the harder it becomes for me to breathe—and we don't go anywhere. The third time, my body somehow, obligingly, agrees to travel to Yugo-Zapadnaya.

At the beginning, Natalya talks with me for a long time. Then, with Little Badger. Then, she invites Little Badger to make up a story and either draw it or enact it using toys. Little Badger happily chooses to play with the toys. The psychologist asks leading questions ("How many people are in your story?" "What are their names?" "Look here, there are so many different dolls and stuffed animals, do you want to choose any of them to be that person?" "How are they related to one another?" "Where do they live?" "How will we dress them?" "What do they want?" and so forth), Sasha makes up a story, and I simply observe. And I feel goosebumps running up my spine. Because you don't need special training in psychology to understand who's who in this tale.

"... Once upon a time there lived two sisters. Two Barbie dolls. They lived in the little Barbie house. The older was named Anna-Maria, she was very beautiful, but not very happy, and she didn't want to be distracted. She wore a big, wide-brimmed hat. The younger sister was named Sandra, and she distracted Anna-Maria from her important thoughts all the time. Then, Anna-Maria pulled her wide-brimmed hat over her face so no one could disturb her while she was thinking about important things. She didn't want to listen to her younger sister Sandra, because she didn't know that Sandra also wanted to tell her something important."

"What important thing?" asks Natalya.

"... She wanted to warn Anna-Maria about danger."

"Danger that specifically threatens Anna-Maria?"

"... Danger that threatens them all. It's a very big danger. A total catastrophe. Their whole family."

"And who are the other members of the family?"

"... They also had an older brother. Here he is... Ken. I generally can't stand Barbie and Ken, but you don't have any other dolls here. So, let this be him. He was named Big. He was also very busy. And they also had a younger brother."

"How old was the younger brother?"

"... The younger brother wasn't any years old. He was very little. He'd just been born."

"And what was his name?"

"He didn't have a name. They hadn't been able to name him yet."

"There are all kinds of baby dolls in that box. Do you want to choose one to be the younger brother?"

"... There's no one there who can be the younger brother. None of them are right. None of those baby dolls will work."

"What should we do about that?"

"... Well, we'll just know that there was also a little brother in the house."

"Maybe we'll put in a crib for him? Look there, in that box—it has children's furniture."

"... No, none of these cribs is right. They won't work. Let's just play as if the little brother who didn't have a name or a crib lived in the house with the sisters. Can we play that way?"

"Of course. You can play any way you want. So, what about the danger that threatened this family?"

"... Next to the house where the sisters lived was a market. On Sundays, the sisters drove to the market in that stupid, pink Barbie car. Actually, their car was a different color, but you don't have that color, so let it be pink... And at the market, a woman worked selling fruit, but actually she was a wicked witch. Also, an alien from another planet. Here, this rag doll with buttons instead of eyes. And she was plotting something very bad..."

"What was she plotting?"

"... That witch wanted to sell Anna-Maria an enchanted apple from another planet disguised as healthy food. So that Anna-Maria would take the apple home. And inside the apple sat a piece of the witch herself. The witch planned to crawl out of the apple and steal the baby from the house. She knew that if she kidnapped the baby, it would be the end of the world. And the whole earth would perish."

"Why would those things happen after the kidnapping?"

"... Because he was a special baby. Who should never, ever be taken out of the house, for any reason."

One of the center employees looks cautiously through the office door. She gestures that our hour is up, and another child is waiting in the corridor. Our psychologist tenses noticeably.

"We can't stop right now," she says. "That would be a very bad idea. Let them wait. We still need a little time."

The employee frowns slightly and closes the door.

"That means that the wicked witch wanted to destroy the whole earth?"

"... Yes. Because she came from another planet."

"But the younger sister, Sandra, guessed her treacherous plans."

"... Yes, Sandra immediately saw that the fruit seller was a real witch. And she asked Anna-Maria not to buy any apples from her, but Anna-Maria didn't listen, she was thinking about something else."

"But Sandra probably thought up a way to warn her older sister about the danger?"

"... She never managed to do that. Every time Sandra wanted to warn her, Anna-Maria pulled her hat over her face."

"And then Sandra had an idea? Some way to do it? She was very quick-witted. And resourceful. As soon as she guessed that the fruit seller was a terrible witch, then she probably had an idea about what to do with the hat?"

"... The younger sister was smart, yes. But she chattered too much. And therefore, no one guessed how smart she was. And no one listened to her."

"But did she know that she was very smart?"

"... Well, she wasn't certain."

"Maybe she convinced herself when she found a way to fix things with the wicked witch? She fixed things, then, at the market?"

"... Yes. Sandra fixed things with the wicked witch. She found a way. When Anna-Maria was preparing to take the apple from the witch's hand, Sandra grabbed the hat off her head and flung it at the witch. It was so unexpected that the witch turned from a fruit seller into the alien monster she really was. And Anna-Maria couldn't pull the hat over her face and screen herself from everything. Therefore, she also saw that the fruit seller was an alien monster. And then she even thanked Sandra for her help. And they went home."

"Very good. Now we can say goodbye until next time." The psychologist turns to me. "Please bring your husband with you."

She refuses to take money for the visit. She smiles.

"This is a free center. Don't be embarrassed. Sometimes, you just need to accept help."

The next time—the second and last, as the center closes for the summer holidays—Natalya talks very little with Little Badger. She gives her several pretty colored pebbles ("This orange one—let it be your happiness. When you feel sad, squeeze it in your hand. And this lilac one is your confidence in yourself. If you doubt your intelligence or your beauty, take it in your hand, this way... And this blue one is your strength. If you feel sick, choose it..."). And then she sends Little Badger to leaf through books and draw, and she talks with us.

She wants to be sure I understand who my daughter identified with in that play story, who I was, and so forth. I say, of course, I understand. After all, even the names were telling us something. Sasha is Sandra. I am Anna-Maria. The little brother for whom none of the baby dolls will work—that's understood. And everything's clear with the witch—it's sorrow, it's danger, it's death, in fact. But why are we all sisters and brothers? I, my husband, she herself, and our dead baby?

She says this is a very typical displacement. Slightly different names. A slightly different family arrangement. Making up this story, a child simply pours out her anxiety, not understanding that this story is about us. Although, of course, it is in fact about us.

I ask if I understand correctly that Sasha's complaints about her health are a kind of attention seeking, an attempt to tear off the "wide-brimmed hat" with which I fence myself off, but she answers that that's not it.

Of course, she says, the child is missing some attention, and it wouldn't be a bad thing to share some "special time" with her, but that's not the main thing. The main thing is that she's trying to help me. She's trying to take part of my problem on herself, part of the responsibility. She sees it's hard for me to breathe and intuitively, as much as she can, tries to share that with me. And she says it's hard for her to breathe, too. She isn't making it up. She really feels that way. But, all the same, she's a child. She shouldn't take responsibility for me: my husband and I need to unburden her of that.

"But how?" asks my husband.

She draws a picture with a ballpoint pen: two boats, a big one and a little one, and a dock with a wooden piling. The boats are tied to the piling. She says:

"This piling—that's you, Alexander. And these boats are your wife and daughter. Now, they're holding onto you. They don't have any other support. That's not right. This big boat must float independently again. Then, the little boat will also float. But if this big boat is uncoupled from you now, it will simply be carried away by the current. Right now, there's no one in control of it." She turns to me. "You need help. Professional psychological help. When your daughter sees that they can really help you and that she isn't responsible for you, she will immediately get better."

"And could you help me? I like the way you work."

She sighs:

"I work with children. In some ways, it's simpler with children than with adults. They're able to endure and overcome difficult situations through play, to heal through play. Adults can't do that."

She says I need a professional who's able to work with loss. Particularly, the loss of a child. But she doesn't personally know any such professional. She does know a psychologist who works with panic attacks—but that's not exactly what's needed.

She says goodbye and wishes us luck. And promises that Little Badger will certainly be better after these two sessions.

CHAPTER 21
THE BOTTOM

The end of May. Little Badger really is better. She doesn't complain about her health any more, and we send her to Riga to visit her grandmother and grandfather.

The two of us remain, Sasha and I. The wooden piling and the rotting boat tied to it, which has sprung a leak. If the boat comes untied from that piling, the current won't even carry it away. It won't float anywhere. It'll simply sink to the bottom.

On one of the first days of summer, I discover what the bottom looks like. I get outside after almost a week of sitting at home and walk to the school where Little Badger is a student to retrieve a forgotten pair of shoes. It's a ten-minute walk from home to the school. I walk about twenty minutes. But I don't get to the school. I have literally only around twenty yards left—but I just can't get there. My heart pounds, my head swims, my breath catches, my skin goes numb—just the way it always happens, only ten times worse than usual. I see a bench on the boulevard, it's only a couple of steps to the bench—but I can't take them. It seems I'm dying. I sit down, right there on the ground. Right on top of candy wrappers, sunflower seed husks, drops of ice cream, pigeon dung, dust. On Usachyov Street. Next to a garbage bin.

People walk around me in a wide arc. A woman grabs the hand of a small child and quickly leads him away. A man in sweats nervously calls a lop-eared puppy who's rushed to lick my hand. Too bad. Such a fine puppy. I didn't get to pet him.

I poke at my cell phone with frozen fingers, but the touch screen refuses to recognize my skin as human. On the tenth attempt, I somehow manage to call my husband.

I tell him I'm sitting on the ground next to a garbage bin and a bench on Usachyov Street, and that I think I'm dying.

He answers:

"Don't be afraid. I'll come get you, right now."

He walks towards me for ten minutes, continuing to talk with me on the cell phone the whole way. Because it seems to me that if I stop hearing his voice, the rope that's already come loose and no longer keeps me on the surface next to the piling will snap in two—and that I'll remain at the bottom forever.

He arrives and pulls me back from the bottom. He literally carries me in his arms. In a couple of minutes, I'm better, and he puts me down. I walk on my own. I breathe. I feel my body. I'm at the dock again.

But now I know exactly what the bottom looks like.

The kind of bottom where a good owner won't let his puppy go.

The kind of bottom from which no one, except Sasha, can bring me back.

Chapter 22
Treatment Required

After that incident, I decide that I really do need professional help. Not some un-known lady who's taken some unknown psychology courses after her divorce (I'd already met a couple of those—they were useless), but a regular state institution where trained professionals work.

I turn to the Clinic for Nervous Disorders on Rossolimo Street. I arrive for an appointment with a neurologist. I describe my trouble with swallowing, breath-ing, panic attacks, rapid heartbeat, sleeplessness. I explain the back story. I ask the neurologist to prescribe antidepressants—or whatever else is customary in such circumstances.

"You need a good psychologist," says the neurologist.

"To this point, I haven't been able to find one who can help me."

"That's just because you were looking in the wrong place!" answers the neurol-ogist, cheerfully. "You probably turned to private practices. To so-called specialists who've got certificates from who knows where and now just take your money."

"Where should I have looked?"

"What do you mean, where? We have them right here."

"You have psychologists here?"

"Of course! A whole floor of psychologists. All are outstanding specialists. You're registered in Moscow and have an insurance card? Excellent! In that case, the appointment's absolutely free. Have a seat, make yourself comfortable in the corridor for now. I'll call the psychologists and find out who can see you, and I'll take you there immediately."

"What, right now?"

"Well, of course. Your situation's urgent. You practically don't eat, you're losing weight..."

As I make myself comfortable in the corridor, I'm almost happy. Finally. Help is coming. A whole floor of free, professional psychologists—exactly what I need. And I've wasted all this time for nothing!

The neurologist and I go up to another floor. For some reason, the door to the psychology department is locked. The neurologist rings the bell. After a couple of minutes, a gloomy, copper-haired lady who looks like the childcare worker from my creepiest kindergarten memories silently opens the door. It smells like kindergarten on the psychology floor, too—like rag mops and boiled cabbage. The child-care lady lets us onto the floor, silently locks the door from inside, and puts the key in her pocket.

The neurologist leads me along a melancholy yellow corridor. I ask if there's a bathroom and, stopping short, she points to a door at the far end. For some reason, the bathroom is also like the one at kindergarten. White tile. The toilets are separated from one another with low partitions. There are no doors. None at all. On a tile podium next to the toilets, there's a dilapidated bathtub with a dirty-grey curtain. I try to imagine what use that bathtub is to a client coming for an appointment with a professional psychologist, but my imagination fails.

I return to the neurologist; she leads me to a little nook in front of some kind of unnamed office and asks me to sit on the bench. I'm liking the psychology department less and less, but I sit, out of politeness. You never know, after all. Perhaps they just have this Soviet way of doing things but the psychologists are actually excellent. It really could be that way, if you think about it.

The neurologist sticks her head into the office and quietly says something to an unseen psychologist. Then, she closes the door and turns to me:

"So, everything's arranged. Wait right here. She'll call you soon."

I wait. Next to me on the bench sits a woman in a garish gown and worn-out slippers who's also waiting for the psychologist to call her. The woman is constantly brushing her hair. With her hand. More precisely, as if she has a comb in place of her hand. She combs her greasy hair back. Then, forward. Then, she parts it. And then, she combs it back again. Her chart lies on her knees. On the front are her last name, first name, patronymic, date of birth. And her diagnosis: MDP. Manic-depressive psychosis.

I look at the lady in the gown combing her hair, and I think about the toilets without doors, about the locked door to the floor, and also that the term "psychologist" is obviously used in a very broad sense in the Clinic for Nervous Disorders. My thoughts are interrupted by the voice of the psychologist:

"Anna Starobinets? Come in."

The psychologist is a stern beauty with skillfully drawn-on eyebrows, about twenty-five years old.

"So, I understand you have problems with taking food?"

I begin to tell her about the pregnancy, about childhood polycystic kidney disease, about induced childbirth—but she isn't interested in any of that. She's interested in food. In why, exactly, I'm not able to eat.

"So, you see food. How do you feel when you see it? What do you think?"

"About what?"

"About the food?"

"Nothing."

"Nothing at all? Or maybe you think that the food's unpleasant? Does the food disgust you?"

"No."

"But you don't have any appetite, either?"

"Not especially."

"Does it seem to you that the food's not fresh? Or poisoned?"

"No, absolutely not."

"But what kind of feeling keeps you from eating it?"

"The feeling that I can't swallow it. It's a mechanical issue. Making my throat swallow."

"Did you do a gastroscopy? Did they find anything?"

"Yes, I did. And they didn't find anything."

"That's very good news. But let's return to food. How long have you had this problem with taking food?"

"A couple of months."

"But you manage to eat something?"

"Something."

"How? If you say you can't swallow food?"

"Well, in a few situations, I can."

"Which ones?"

"For example, after I take a drink of strong alcohol. And also—immediately after I wake up. Therefore, recently I've been eating once a day—immediately after I wake up. Right there in bed."

She leans on her arms:

"What do you do, take food to bed with you?"

"No. When I wake up, my husband brings me food."

"Food? Your husband?" she asks again.

"Yes, my husband brings me food."

"In bed?"

"In bed."

"Your husband doesn't work?" She obviously doesn't believe me. Really, what painful fantasies these are—a husband bringing someone food in bed!...

"My husband works at home."

"As what?!"

"A screenwriter. A journalist. A writer."

She makes a note of something in her papers and loses interest in the subject of my husband, who's obviously a figment of my imagination.

"So, you eat once a day—and then it becomes unpleasant for you to take food?"

"And then it continues to be pleasant, but I can't swallow normally."

"Everything's clear. And how do we sleep?"

"It's bad. We have insomnia."

"Understood..." She again writes something, then tears herself away from the papers. "Well, Anna. You need to be hospitalized."

"Why?"

"What do you mean, why? To treat you."

"What do you mean, 'treat' me? How are you proposing to treat me?"

"With various medications."

"Which ones?"

"Well, Anna. Choosing medications is the doctor's job. You don't need to worry about that. Your job is to be hospitalized and treated, without worrying about anything..."

She's very young. Younger than I am. Not some relic of punitive Soviet psychiatry. So, where did that intonation come from? That stern expression of her drawn-on eyebrows? That choice of words?

"How can I not worry about what medications are used to treat me?" I ask, tiredly. "This is my health we're talking about. Not knowing how you plan to treat me, I won't be able to make a decision."

"What decision?"

"About being hospitalized."

She looks at me as if I'm a space alien, with a green tentacle on my forehead.

"All right, if it's so important to you—you'll receive tranquilizers, antidepressants, and antipsychotics, both intravenously and orally. Do you understand any of that?"

"Yes, I understand everything."

"That's good. Plan on three to four weeks. I'll admit you now. Have some of your relatives bring you..."

"No, thank you."

"What?"

"Thank you, I don't want to be hospitalized for three or four weeks."

"How can that be—you don't want to? Why?"

"First of all, I work."

"You work?! As what?!"

"A screenwriter. And a writer."

"But you just said it's your husband..."

"It's me, as well. But this isn't just about work. I simply, absolutely, don't want to receive intravenous and oral tranquilizers, antidepressants, and antipsychotics."

"But what do you mean by saying 'I don't want to,' Anna? You and I aren't children. There's no such thing as 'I don't want to.' You require hospitalization—that means that you have to be hospitalized. You have an eating disorder. As a doctor, I'm responsible for you. I don't have the right to send you home in this condition."

I feel like a character in some kind of film, or story, when a journalist comes to a madhouse to write an article and then suddenly turns out to be the patient—

and the door's locked, and the character's put in a straitjacket, and a nurse stabs a sedative into a vein, saying, gently, 'Well, of course, you're a journalist, a famous journalist, don't worry!' I think about the locked door to the floor. About the toilets without doors. And I'm even slightly afraid. But the confusion, luckily, passes quickly.

"As a journalist, I can assure you that you, as a doctor, have full authority to send me home. In this country, we have compulsory psychiatric treatment only by court order."

"Yes, of course! Go home, whatever you want. Am I forcibly detaining you? You don't have to talk that way. We just want to help you. Goodbye."

"Goodbye. Open the door for me, please."

… But some other woman without a journalist's experience, less grounded in legal questions, or simply more trusting and gullible—that woman might still be there today. Hospitalized. Believing in "a doctor's responsibility." Resigning herself to "you need to means—you need to." Perhaps it might even have helped her. However, I don't believe it. A cocktail of antipsychotics, antidepressants, tranquilizers, disrespect, neglect, and discouragement can't possibly help anyone.

I'm so angry that I reach home without a single panic attack, and at home I eat three sandwiches. In a certain way, the professional psychologist at the Clinic for Nervous Disorders has helped me a great deal. Unfortunately, the therapeutic effect doesn't last long. I don't fall asleep until close to morning, and the day after, I'm again unable to breathe and eat normally.

Chapter 23
Olives and Paradoxes

In the end, I turn to the specialist on panic attacks whom the child psychologist recommended. His name is Alexander, he doesn't have an office, he sees patients at home.

He helps me. I have no idea if he's a professional in good standing or a charlatan, if his methods of psychotherapy were thought out in advance, or whether the stars just aligned. In my case, specifically, he turns out to be absolutely the right person.

He's approaching fifty. He's lean, stoop-shouldered, shy when he meets you, and unsure of himself. He warns that he works with panic attacks and not "loss," so in our case, it's as if he's treating just the symptoms. He tries so hard to be a correct psychotherapist that he literally "tips his hand": he repeats my own phrases after me, slightly reformulating them (in the textbook, apparently, that's called "reflecting emotions back to the patient"), tries not to use negative statements.

He says we'll try to work without pills. He shows me simple but effective breathing exercises for relaxation and lowering my pulse rate (the secret is simple: the exhale must be much longer than the inhale), and also for reducing muscle tension (also simple: to relax the muscles, you first need to tense them as tightly as possible). But these aren't the things with which he helps me the most. It's with his intuition, common sense, ability to look at things from an unusual point of view—and, correspondingly, his freedom from conventional thinking.

For me, Alexander the psychologist plays the role not so much of a psychologist as a clever rabbi who gives paradoxical advice to a sad Jew.

"... I have insomnia."

"You don't sleep well. You need to walk around in the fresh air for a minimum of thirty minutes every day."

"But I can't! That's exactly the problem! I can't walk away from home. As soon as I move away from the building, my panic attacks start."

"Oy. Did I say you have to move away from the building? That's absolutely not required. Walk around the building. If you want, walk back and forth next to the entrance. I don't care. What's important to me is that you, first, walk for thirty minutes, and second, do it in the fresh air."

I start walking around the building—and day by day, I discover that I can walk calmly for thirty minutes, without stopping, at a fairly brisk pace, and absolutely not run out of breath. As soon as I satisfy myself of that, the ability to move away from the building for a minimum distance of a half-hour walk comes back to me. Buying pizza at the Dove Café stops being a problem.

"... I can't swallow food normally. Only in the morning, immediately after I wake up."

"You eat once a day. That seems too little to you."

"Yes!"

"And how many times a day can you drink?"

"As many as I want."

"Then during the day, drink cocoa, sweet tea, a milkshake. Considering your full breakfast, you won't have the slightest chance of starving yourself to death."

I start drinking cocoa and milkshakes. I relax, stop getting hung up, and don't try shoving food into myself during the day anymore just because I have to. And I unexpectedly discover that I'm able to mechanically grab any old piece of food lying around and, without turning on my brain, swallow it without any problem.

"... And what if, in spite of everything, I have some kind of terrible illness? Although I had myself checked out. Cancer, for example. And instead of treating that illness, I'm treating panic attacks."

"You're afraid you have a serious illness. Although the doctors didn't find it. Well, I can't give you any guarantee that you don't have a serious illness. It really does happen that doctors miss things. It might make sense to do some more investigating. That's not my specialty. But you *do* have panic attacks—that's a fact. Even if you have cancer—why do you need panic attacks on top of that?"

I undergo still more medical tests. As before, they don't find any serious illness. But even if they find one, why do I need panic attacks? It's unclear, indeed.

"... My husband's suggesting we go to Greece."

"Your husband wants you to go to Greece. Excellent."

"That's not excellent at all! How can I go anywhere in this condition? When I eat once a day, don't sleep, and continually feel terrible?"

"I don't see any problem. You can absolutely do all of that easily, the same way, in Greece. Eat once a day—but eat feta cheese and olives. Don't sleep—but listen to the waves then. And feel bad. Who said you're required to feel bad only in Russia? You can feel hideous in Greece. It's not forbidden."

"And if something happens to me?"

"You mean in the medical sense?"

"Yes."

"You'll call an ambulance."

We go to Greece. I fall asleep to the sound of the waves. I swim. I write some screenplays. I eat feta cheese and olives. I drink red wine and retsina. I even call an ambulance—because I have a terrible allergic reaction to something I've eaten or drunk. In the midnight ambulance, covered from head to toe in crimson hives, surrounded by a large Greek family taking their harsh, swarthy grandfather to the doctor with a gunshot wound, I feel that I'm alive. And that it's getting easier.

Chapter 24
A Boy

It's a full year after the birth, in winter, before I'm finally better.

In another half-year, in August, I'm pregnant again.

When the ultrasound and blood test confirm the pregnancy, Little Badger constructs a whole row of stuffed animal talismans on the chest of drawers next to my bed. I look into their artificial eyes and experience not the happiness I was expecting to feel, but horror. The trap has sprung. The clock starts ticking. What have I done.

It all happens again. Everything that happened with me last time, literally right up to the season. Who says bad luck doesn't strike twice? It's fall again, rain and mud. It's Little Badger's birthday—and I have morning sickness. The very same excited children, gifts, and a cake with candles, in a nauseous haze. Even Nika, my friend, is expecting, just like she was then. It's as if I'd been carried back in a time machine to two years ago. Except now, I know what comes next.

The weeks will pass. The morning sickness will end. In the wet, November dark, I'll go for an ultrasound, and they'll tell me it's a boy. A silence will hang in the air, and I'll understand that bad luck has struck again.

My friend's baby will be born, and mine won't.

The weeks pass. The morning sickness ends. In the wet, November dark, I go to Dr. Malmberg for an ultrasound.

She says:

"It's a boy."

A silence hangs in the air. Then, she says:

"He has healthy kidneys."

I give birth in April, in Latvia. Because in Moscow, thanks to my high blood pressure and pulse, I'm supposed to give birth only in a specialized maternity hospital for women with cardiology problems. Visiting hours there are from three to five in the afternoon—and women with high blood pressure are not permitted to have a husband present at the birth or after the birth. In the Jūrmala maternity hospital, they don't see any connection between high blood pressure and a husband's presence.

... Full dilation of the cervix. Contractions are beginning. I close my eyes and scream from pain and fear.

Through my own screams, I hear how the midwife is speaking to me, calmly and quietly, with a Latvian accent. She says it's almost over. Very soon, it will be all over. But for that to happen, I have to stop screaming. I have to exhale, then inhale, exhale again, and push. But I don't have to scream. I don't have to.

She says:

"Let him out. You have to let him out, understand?"

I listen to her voice. I exhale, inhale.

I let him out.

"A baby, Anya!" my husband cries, in amazement. "We have a baby... Look at him!"

We have a baby. Funny. Grey-eyed. He smiles and quivers in his sleep. Sometimes, he's afraid of loud noises. Sometimes, he thinks he's losing his balance and falling down. Then, he stretches out his little arms widely and sharply—as if he's trying to open unseen wings into the void. As if he's trying to fly away. And I pick him up and whisper: don't be afraid, don't be afraid. I won't let you go anywhere. I'll look at you.

Afterword

February 2016. We're in Berlin again. My husband, Sasha Garros, is sick. Through social media, we've been able to amass the enormous, unreal amount of money for his treatment, which—that's how the stars aligned—is again taking place at Charité. Radiation and chemotherapy. There's a very difficult operation in January. Our children—eleven-year-old Little Badger and ten-month-old Lyova—are here with us. The treatment goes well, but we don't know what will happen next.

A month after the operation, when Sasha gets better, he and I sit on the U-Bahn and travel to station Kurt-Schumacher-Platz. It's dank and cold on the street, a wide grey avenue, dull grey buildings, frozen grey people getting onto buses at the bus stop. For a long time, we're lost; we wander along the avenue, first in one direction, then in the opposite direction. Finally, we find the right cross street and turn into the quiet little street leading to the Dankes-Nazareth cemetery.

It's an extremely well-cared-for cemetery by a Protestant church. Neat fir and spruce trees grow here. Red squirrels leap about here. Tegel Airport is close by, and every few minutes, planes take off into the sky. Three years ago, strangers saying prayers in a foreign language buried our baby here, in a common grave. We roam around the cemetery and soon find the right place. It's not hard to find the place: it looks like a children's playground constructed among the tombstones.

There's not just one common grave, as we expected: there are fifteen. They're surrounded by a large, neat, empty lawn for new graves. The ones that are here resemble large sandboxes in which children celebrating their birthdays forgot their gifts. Teddy bears, wooden horses, iron birds, kites, porcelain angels, rainbow pinwheels spinning in the wind, flowers, candles, and—carved pebbles. Pebbles with a date of birth that corresponds to the date of death. The more recent the date, the better preserved the gifts. The more distant—the worse preserved.

In our "sandbox," where all the stones indicate 2012–2013, the pinwheels look almost new, and there are many fresh flowers and candles that haven't burned out, but the bears are swollen with rain and have turned grey, while the horses are peeling. A garish, pink owlet on a stick rotates its head with every gust of wind, giving out a squeaky, melancholy moan.

It's possible that they play together there.

It's possible. After all, they have all these toys. All of them, except our baby. He doesn't have any toys, or a stone. Maybe they don't let him play because of that?

"What if they don't share with him?" I say, aloud.

"I don't think so," answers my Sasha, not at all disturbed by the idiotic question. "They're all here forever at the age when there's no understanding of 'mine' and 'yours.' There's no greediness yet, either. I don't think they're unkind."

We look at the stones. *Kleine Kosmonaut*, May 1, 2013. *Unser kleiner Engel*, December 21, 2012. *Wir vermissen dich, Emily.* Little Cosmonaut. Little Angel. We miss you, Emily. We miss you, Kurt. Marta. Thomas.

On a few stones, there are two names. You can calculate the difference between the dates, and it's as if you're reading a story. Here it is, the difference is in the year: one died, after three months they tried again, conceived, gave birth—and the second one also died. And here, a difference of two months: one died immediately, the second suffered a little longer. And here, on this stone: one date for both. Little twins. They were born and died together. Two identical pinwheels are launched simultaneously by a gust of wind.

"All the same, we have to leave him something," I say.

We rummage in our backpacks. When you have children, you always find some kind of toy junk in your backpack. Big Badger finds a tiny, porcelain rabbit with a broken paw. I find a bracelet of rubber bands made by Little Badger. We place the bracelet, the rabbit, and his broken-off paw on the grave. With a roar, an airplane takes off into the sky. Our gift looks pitiful.

"Let's come back here again," says Sasha. "We'll bring him something better. And we'll place a stone."

... I'm in a children's store that looks very much like the one I often dream about. But then again, all children's stores look alike. As in the dream, I'm choosing toys—only now, I know for whom. For two little boys, one living, and one dead. For the living boy, I quickly find what he'll like—a multicolored, roly-poly owlet sewn from pieces of fabric of various textures and colors, with a little bell inside. With the gift for the other boy, I unexpectedly fall into a stupor. It seems like a purely symbolic gesture, I can just take the first toy that falls into my hand... I take one, then another—and simply can't choose. I seriously try to understand what he'll like best of all, what he'll love. I try ten varieties of stuffed animals, I imagine how they'll swell in the spring rain, and I put them back. Who wants to play with a swollen dog? I look at cars, trains, airplanes—none of them is right. Finally, it comes to me that I'm rooting around in the wrong department. He's really small. As small as can be. A newborn. I go to the department for babies and quickly find what I need: a hanging clip-on toy with soft sheep-rattles and multicolored balls and leaves. The kind that hangs on a stroller or over a crib that the baby can see and stretch his hands towards. Upwards, from below.

That's exactly what we need. Because he really is down below. Under the ground.

... We write "Littlest Badger" on the stone, in waterproof marker. And the date beneath, December 13, 2012—the day of birth and death. We light a candle in a special metal housing. We stick a rainbow pinwheel into the ground. Attach the clip-on toy. The wind immediately spins the multicolored blades, tugs at the sheep and blows them around, blows on the candle—not enough to blow it out, but enough to make the flame tremble. A plane takes off into the sky with a roar that won't wake anyone up.

During the last week, a new grave has appeared on the spacious lawn. It isn't yet enclosed with a stone border, and the earth's still quite loose. On it are fresh flowers, a pair of porcelain angels, and a pile of children's things in the very smallest size —colored onesies, a blanket with bears, a cap, and socks. They'd prepared a layette for the maternity hospital—and brought it to the cemetery.

... In our rented Berlin apartment, our son Lyova meets us. Tangled up in his trousers and smacking his palms on the parquet floor, he crawls into the hallway on all fours, stops still for a second—and smiles from puppy-like happiness at seeing us. He smiles over his whole face—with drooling gums; shining eyes; the whitish down of eyebrow; an impudent button nose; and fat, round cheeks. I hold out the roly-poly owlet to Lyova, and he cautiously accepts my gift.

Fascinated, he looks at the toy, feeling the velvety red beak and back, striped cotton wings, corduroy head with white polka dots, the silk breast with blue flowers, the linen stomach in green check, the knitted blue scarf. He freezes in amazement every time his fingers come across the seams between pieces. He points to where the strange bird's eyes are. He listens to the sound of the bell hidden in the rag belly of the owlet. He gurgles, pants, and frowns, trying to lay the roly-poly owlet on its back, to grasp its marvelous secret, to understand why it won't be conquered.

In the Berlin church cemetery, the pink owlet on a stick gives out its squeaky, melancholy sound with every gust of wind. In the Berlin church cemetery, red squirrels leap about. In the Berlin church cemetery, every baby has gifts and a stone—and ours does, too. Planes fly over the Berlin church cemetery.

And soon, we'll find ourselves on one of these planes. And taking off, I'll hug my son to myself and look down through the window. I'm afraid of heights, but I'll look, all the same.

I'll look at him.

2013–2016

PART TWO

OTHERS

ADVANCE WARNING

When the publisher's staff read my manuscript, it seemed to them that a first-person confessional narrative, meaning my personal story, might not be enough for Russian readers. That it wouldn't hurt the book to add one additional section: interviews with doctors, psychologists, and other women who'd lost children. Although I resisted a bit, in the end I concluded that they were right. And I decided to add another few parts to the book, more journalistic than literary, that have a more applied, practical purpose. Women who are experiencing loss and the medical personnel (doctors, midwives, psychologists) who work with them will find useful information here, and a bit of not-uninteresting advice, and examples of a different kind of medical and human experience.

In general, in this section I very much wanted to initiate something like a dialogue among Russian women and Russian doctors, summoning this last group to the conversation. I had questions for the German specialists concerning their experience but, naturally, questions most of all for Russian doctors. Has anything changed in their approach to late termination of pregnancy over the last few years? Have other methods of termination been adopted, what kind of anesthesia is used, are relatives permitted to be present, is psychological help being offered to mothers, is saying goodbye to the baby allowed? What ethical principles are medical personnel guided by? Are there psychological studies and various types of statistics on this issue? Is there any understanding that the existing system is cruel, and is there any wish to change it?

Unfortunately, that dialogue didn't happen. As open as the German health care system was to me—a woman who'd undergone the termination of such a pregnancy and the author of a book documenting it—the Russian system was just as closed. To put it bluntly, it wasn't possible for me to talk with Moscow doctors working in this field. I wasn't able to talk with anyone at either the Infectious Diseases Clinical Hospital No. 2 in Sokolinaya Gora or at the Kulakov Research Center for Obstetrics, Gynecology, and Perinatology on Oparin Street, where they now perform late termination of pregnancy. At the hospital in Sokolinaya Gora, I was informed that they'd speak with me only if ordered to do so by the Moscow Department of Health; at the Kulakov Center, they simply ignored my request.

I might have been able to get to them through the "back door," might have tried to find ways to approach doctors willing to answer my questions off the record, without giving their names or job titles, through my acquaintances. I might have been able to do that, but I chose not to. It seems to me that the situation I've described reflects reality best of all, and that it so graphically demonstrates the difference in approaches that nothing more is needed. On the one hand, we have the German system, plainly oriented towards the individual (and in that system, even extremely busy doctors occupying important positions respond promptly to my request for an interview because they believe it's right to "spread the word about this subject in Russia"). And on the other hand, we have the Russian system —closed off to the individual under lock and key.

And here we have people—unfortunate women, stubborn women, brave women, and sometimes their men, who are trying to break through those locks.

I hope that sooner or later we succeed.

CB   BD

Thanks to Berlin journalist Elena Jerzdeva for help in organizing interviews with German medical personnel; to the doctors of the Charité-Virchow Obstetrical Clinic for their openness and for finding time for me; and to the Russian mamas who've lost children, for their strength of spirit, and for their willingness to tell their stories in my book.

Ultrasound Doctor

Wolfgang Henrich, Doctor of Medicine, Professor (Berlin)

"That fetus has human rights"

Professor Henrich is a doctor of medicine, director of the Charité-Virchow Obstetrical Clinic, and head of the Department of Ultrasound Diagnostics. In the hierarchy of the profession, he ranks no lower than the deputy head doctor for Obstetrics and Gynecological Care of the hospital in Sokolinaya Gora. He doesn't speak Russian. He doesn't live in Russia. He's a very busy person. However, agreeing with him about an interview for my book is considerably easier than with the deputy head doctor of the Moscow hospital. He doesn't need an order from any ministry to do this—just his own goodwill.

Let's say you perform an ultrasound on a pregnant woman, she's lying happily in front of you and impatiently waiting for news: girl or boy? And you see that something's not right with the fetus, something serious. How do you conduct yourself in such a situation?

When I discover some kind of defect, it's very important for me to continue the study, to attentively examine the fetus from head to toe. If you're an experienced doctor, you usually see the defect in the first ten to twenty seconds of the exam. But in that situation, it's even more important to conduct a full exam because there's the risk of missing something important. For example, when you find a heart defect, it's very important not to fixate on just the heart but to examine the whole body, because if some fetal pathology besides the heart defect is revealed, that immediately, significantly, raises the risk of a chromosomal abnormality. If the heart defect is isolated, the risk of some sort of syndrome or a pathological karyotype is low. If you inform the woman of your findings immediately, you won't have the chance to continue and finish the study because the mother will be very worried, frightened, she'll ask questions and distract you. Even if they send me a woman where some sort of birth defect is already suspected, I conduct a full and thorough study. I have to concentrate. There must be empathy between doctor and patient, and I always try to engage with the mother, but it's still very important not to start explaining anything about illness and its consequences to her in the middle of the study, because then it will be very difficult to focus simultaneously on both the study and the patient and her reactions. Therefore, I always say to her: "Allow me to examine the baby from head to toe. When I'm finished, I'll tell you everything I've seen and what I think about my findings."

What kind of birth defects do you discover most often by ultrasound?

Most often, problems with the heart. Some 0.8 percent (eight out of one thousand) of all newborns have heart defects, but one-third of them are simple ventricular septal defects, nothing serious. In second place after the heart—one instance in one thousand—are problems with the kidneys and neurological defects. In terms of chromosomal abnormalities, here we have one in five hundred fetuses with Down's Syndrome, that's trisomy of the twenty-first chromosome. Then comes trisomy of the eighteenth chromosome—Edwards Syndrome (one in three thousand). Then trisomy of the thirteenth chromosome, Patau Syndrome (one in five thousand). In total, around 96 percent of all pregnancies develop normally, and in 4 percent we can expect defects. Of that 4 percent, 1.6 percent are various chromosomal anomalies, 1 percent are monogenic congenital defects, and the remainder are sporadic cases caused by infection, metabolic abnormalities, etc.

And my defect? In my case, at first it was assumed that the fetus had autosomal recessive polycystic kidney disease; later, it was determined to be bilateral multicystic dysplastic kidney.

Autosomal recessive polycystic kidney disease is a very rare illness, one case in forty thousand. The kidneys are very large, with a specific echogenic pattern, they practically don't produce urine. As a result, the fetal bladder is empty, a shortage of amniotic fluid develops, and then an absence of amniotic fluid, which leads to hypoplasia (underdevelopment) of the lungs and compression of the chest. The lack of water leads to shortening of the arms and legs, and the face becomes flat (Potter face). Purely theoretically, individual cases of survival are possible with this diagnosis: if the baby is able to breathe after birth, she might receive peritoneal dialysis and then, after the first year of life, perhaps a kidney transplant can be performed. But the problem with this disease is that it usually involves other organs as well, so it's considered fatal. The diagnosis usually comes in the region of twenty weeks. From the perspective of the ultrasound, the cysts are so small that they're hard to distinguish, therefore, polycystic kidney disease is also called "salt and pepper kidneys." In the case of multicystic dysplastic kidney, the cysts look more like berries. There's a good prognosis for survival with multicystic dysplastic kidney, but only if just one kidney is affected, which is most often the case. Bilateral multicystic dysplastic kidney is encountered fairly rarely.

So, you discover a defect—common or rare. You've made a full examination from head to toe. How do you tell a woman the bad news?

I say to her: "Unfortunately, I have to tell you that the news is not very good. Your baby has this or that problem." Then, I emphasize that, besides the defect I've seen, all the remaining organs have developed normally. For example, that the head is in good shape, the abdominal cavity, the arms and legs are also in good shape. But let's say, for example, that there's a problem with the heart. Then, I offer to describe the normal anatomy of the heart for her, and after that what, exactly, developed abnormally in the heart of her baby and what the consequences are. After that, I suggest that the woman consult a specialist. If something isn't right with the heart, I'll call a pediatric cardiologist; if it's something with the abdominal wall, I'll ask a pediatric abdominal surgeon to come. If it's something to do with the brain, I'll ask someone from the Center for Social Pediatrics to tell the mother about anticipated problems with intellectual development. If it's a problem with the brain of a surgical kind, I'll call a children's neurosurgeon. So, these mothers and their partners who might also be present receive an interdisciplinary consultation here, on the territory of the perinatal center. It's important that I don't send patients for consultation anywhere beyond the confines of the center—I invite the specialists here. We sit down together, I demonstrate my findings—I repeat the patient ultrasound for them or show them the recording. Then, we discuss the case and answer the parents' questions.

As a matter of fact, I'd planned to speak not with Professor Henrich, but with Professor Kalache, who confirmed my diagnosis at Charité in 2012 and gave the referral for termination. But Kalache no longer works at the clinic and has left Germany altogether, therefore I had to turn to Henrich, a man I didn't know.

Henrich doesn't resemble Kalache, a gentle and soulful person (at the very least, a person who gives that impression). As a type, he more closely resembles the anesthesiologist Kai—precise, tough, matter-of-fact. He carves out an hour of time for me and finishes the conversation just as that hour runs out. He spouts statistics and cites paragraphs of German law from memory, not stopping for a second to think about things. He speaks in an even voice, and only once during our entire conversation does he demonstrate any kind of human emotion. Does he, for this reason, seem to me to be a specimen of "soulless doctor"? No. The perfect little example of that for me was and remains nice, intelligent, elderly Professor Demidov. Because for nice Professor Demidov, communication with me as a human being ends at the moment of diagnosis—and for dry Professor Henrich, communication with me as a human being starts there. Because Professor Demidov called a group of students to watch my ultrasound, and Professor Henrich would have invited a neonatologist and a nephrologist. Because after the ultrasound, Professor Demidov directed me to go to the gynecological clinic, and Professor Henrich would have sent me to a psychologist. Because Professor Demidov doesn't deal with "those things," and Professor Henrich does. Because Professor Henrich has that same "ethical protocol" at his disposal, and Professor Demidov has only a medical one.

But not because one of these people lacks a soul and the other has one—no. In this case, their souls are of no importance.

What kinds of questions do parents have?

For example: "Is there any guarantee that the mental impairment won't be too serious?" "Can you tell us the survival rate in our case?" "Is an operation possible?" In a few cases, we can predict whether an operation might be carried out and to what degree it would help (for example, the stomach and intestines often work completely normally after an operation), whether the baby will need a wheel chair or will be able to walk on her own. Every case is individual, and we always try to predict the outcome for the child so that the mother can decide whether to keep the baby or not.

Do you have any kind of statistics concerning these decisions—to continue or terminate the pregnancy on the discovery of birth defects?

If there's a chance to avoid disability, or if the risk of permanent disability is low, the majority of women choose to keep the baby and then treat him. If the risk of permanent disability is high, especially in cases of intellectual disability or a serious heart ailment, such as left hypoplasia syndrome, the majority of mothers prefer to terminate the pregnancy. German law, paragraph 218, part 2, states that if the health of the mother is subject to risk as a result of pregnancy or the birth of a disabled child, if her physical or psychological health might suffer as a result, then that pregnancy may be terminated in the interests of the mother's health.

And who makes the decision about whether the psychological health of the patient is at risk?

The patient makes that decision. Not the doctor. This is very important. The doctor must offer options, and we always have two options, even if the defect is fatal, as in your case. All the same, we give the woman the possibility of prolonging the pregnancy, giving birth the natural way, and spending, say, a few hours with the baby. And then, the baby dies. We let them know in advance that we'll take care of the mother and baby while he lives, but that we won't resuscitate him, intubate him, and so forth, that we'll allow him to go. This means that we'll care for the woman during pregnancy, then midwives and doctors will attend the birth, and then the neonatologist will give the baby palliative care, so that he can die peacefully. A few patients say: "No, I don't want to go down that road, I can't continue the pregnancy if the baby is doomed all the same, I want to terminate." In that case, we convene a council, an ethics commission considers the particular case, and when we come to a resolution—this one is a resolution by doctors—that the wish to terminate the pregnancy is reasonable, we inform the mother of our agreement and then give her a minimum of three additional days to think about it. After three working days, another doctor—not the one who made the diagnosis—confirms the diagnosis and schedules the termination. This guarantees that, at the very least, two doctors are involved in making the decision.

Are there any kinds of special ethical aspects of late termination of pregnancy for medical reasons?

There's a very important moment. If the fetus is no older than twenty-one weeks of gestation and we simply induce labor, in 100 percent of cases, he will die naturally because at this stage, his lungs aren't yet able to breathe. In a case like yours, where there's no amniotic fluid, the baby's lungs are even more underdeveloped. So, these babies die in the birth canal or immediately after birth. They might have a heartbeat—but not the ability to breathe. Therefore, in such cases there's no need to carry out feticide—killing the fetus—inside the uterus. Some people do it, but it's not required. If we're talking about pregnancy after twenty-two weeks, from the legal point of view, it's necessary for the doctor to perform feticide, that is, in fact, to kill the baby inside the uterus before the start of contractions or the rupture of the fetal sac. If contractions have already begun or the fetal sac has already ruptured, from the point of view of German law, the birth has already begun. And from the moment birth has begun, the fetus is already a person, from the legal point of view. A person! A person may not be killed.

How is feticide carried out?

There are two methods. One is to inject liquid into the amniotic sac that blocks the fetal heartbeat, usually this is digoxin. The baby swallows the medicine, her heart stops beating, and she dies. The second method is to introduce the drug straight into the umbilical cord. Then it's carried through the veins to the baby's heart and stops it.

Is it quick?

Yes, it's quick. But it's very... direct. We aren't certain which method is more acceptable for the mother from the psychological point of view.[1] As a matter of fact, we need to conduct research in this area on what is more psychologically acceptable for the mother in this very painful situation. For me, feticide—is always very difficult. Not only for the mother, but also for the doctor, if he has human feelings, it's a very painful moment. Nevertheless, sometimes we're compelled to help the mother and perhaps even the fetus go through this.

Under which option does the fetus suffer less?

We don't know. The fetus begins to feel pain somewhere around the twenty-first or twenty-second week, not before. Because as far as I know, the neurons and axions begin to develop at precisely this stage and, correspondingly, the feeling of pain. I don't know what's easier. I'm not a fetus, and I don't have the means to acquire that experience. No one really knows what feelings a fetus experiences at twenty-one weeks and which is more painful—to receive a fatal injection in the heart, or an arrhythmia and heart attack, or to die of suffocation at the moment of birth. How is it possible to conduct research in this field?! That is... I mean to say... how is it possible to obtain this knowledge?

... For the first time in our entire conversation, Professor Henrich begins to speak nervously and loses his train of thought. Dismay and vexation are in his eyes. I'd put a question to him—and he'd clearly put the question to himself more than once—for which no answer exists. There are not and cannot be any statistics, any laws, any scientific methods of measuring the depths of this human pain. In the post-operative rooms of the Charité clinic hang special reminders with a pain scale and the words: "Dear patient! You don't have to suffer from severe pain. If you're in pain, inform medical personnel about it; modern medicines allow a person to be relieved of pain. Rate the intensity of your pain on a scale of zero to ten. The goal is for you not to be in pain, or to be in very little pain." But a fetus—or shall we call

---

[1] Meaning termination involving feticide or without feticide.

her a baby?—can never give Professor Henrich a number. Her suffering isn't measured on a ten-point scale... The professor quickly masters himself and returns to a neutral tone:

I want to say: it's a very painful situation for everyone involved, no one among the doctors likes to do a termination. But sometimes, we have to do it in order to help the mother. And if we're doing it, we have to provide her with psychological support.

What kind of support do you mean?

It's very important that the parents have a chance to see the baby, if they want to. It's important that the fetus is in fact a dead human, a person. That fetus has human rights—for example, to receive a name and a grave, including a personal grave. Then, it's important to offer the parents a whole range of medical research that will help them understand the reason for the birth defect. Besides that, the woman has to have the chance to receive psychological help afterwards. For such mothers, it's very important to talk about their problem, it's easier for them to find peace and to reconcile themselves with their misfortune. It might be needed weeks or months later. Perhaps one of the reasons you're writing a book about your loss is because for you, it's a means to psychologically overcome what's happened.

Possibly.

Yes. Therefore, you work on a book. Therefore, you've come back here to Charité. And therefore, you're conducting an interview with me now.

Are many unable to "find peace"? How many pregnancies are terminated every year for medical reasons?

In Germany, around two thousand pregnancies are terminated every year as a result of a prenatal diagnosis.[2] But you must know that there are another two hundred thousand terminations a year—those are terminations of completely healthy babies, ordinary abortions "for social reasons" between six and eleven weeks.[3] Women become pregnant by accident, it doesn't matter to them whether the fetus is healthy or not, they just don't want it. That

---

[2] In the table of statistics that Dr. Klapp sent me, this number is higher.

[3] In the table of statistics, this number, on the other hand, is almost two times lower.

is, only 1 percent of all terminations are for medical reasons. I'm certain the situation's similar in Russia.

How do you feel about this situation?

Well, in this case, I find myself in a comfortable situation because at Charité, we don't terminate healthy pregnancies at any stage at all. In the university clinic, terminations are performed only if there's a risk to the health of the mother, if the pregnancy occurred as the result of rape, or if there's a serious fetal pathology.

Do you terminate in the case of Down's Syndrome?

If a woman wants to terminate such a pregnancy, first we send her for a consultation with a psychologist and a doctor-geneticist. Then, we suggest that she meet with a pediatrician who can tell her about such children, and also meet with families in which there are children with Down's Syndrome. After that, the woman is given a minimum of three working days to think about it, and if she still wants to terminate the pregnancy because of Down's Syndrome, yes, we do that. But first, we make sure that there's no conflict between the parents because of the decision, that both are agreed and certain in their decision, that the decision hasn't been made because they're frightened or in a hurry. Haste is very bad for making good decisions. We tell them that they have enough time. That they can calmly take even a few more days to make the decision. Because it's important to make a decision that they can both live with for the rest of their lives.

There are many patient-immigrants in your clinic from various countries that have various cultural codes and religious views. Does everyone make the same decision in the same situation?

No, the decisions are different. For example, Muslims and a few Catholics refuse to terminate pregnancy for religious reasons. Especially Muslims. They say: "We'll accept any child." Even in the case of Down's Syndrome, they say: "Allah sent us this child, and we don't have the right to terminate his life." I'm now caring for two couples expecting a baby with Down's Syndrome. In one case, the patient has known her diagnosis since the tenth week—and she chose to continue the pregnancy all the same, even though the pregnancy was at such an early stage. In the tenth week, she underwent a non-invasive test (that's an analysis of the mother's blood, it became available in the last four years, and it allows us to detect Down's Syndrome in 99.8 percent of cases), then, during the ultrasound, I saw a few markers—but she decided to carry the pregnancy to term. So now, she's already at thirty weeks, and she'll give birth to that baby. And she and her husband are really, completely happy. It's interesting that they didn't even do an amniocentesis—and only it can give a 100-percent, guaranteed result—so as not to harm the baby as a result of the procedure. And the other couple did the amniocentesis, which confirmed Down's Syndrome, and the baby also has a heart defect—but they also decided to give birth to the child. But these couples are, of course, in the minority. The majority of patients terminate a pregnancy with Down's Syndrome, especially if the diagnosis is early, in the region of thirteen weeks, and friends and relatives might not yet even know about the pregnancy. If the diagnosis is made after twenty-three to twenty-four weeks, then the parents often say: "It's too far along, the baby's already big, we'll carry her to term."

Diagnostic methods improve quickly these days; it's possible to find various abnormalities much earlier. Where will this lead?

From the perspective of a fetus with Down's Syndrome, for example, early diagnosis is not beneficial. Because if the truth comes to light later rather than sooner, the baby will have a chance to survive. From the mother's perspective, if the syndrome is discovered early, she may terminate the pregnancy with less psychological and medical trauma for herself. Our ethical system is such that, in the case of a conflict of interest between fetus and mother, the mother has the decisive right to choose. And she may employ it against her own fetus.

PATIENT NO. 1

Zhanna, mother of Yegor (Moscow)

"Come back by nine tomorrow, and don't give it a thought"

In 2014, during the seventeenth week of pregnancy, Zhanna heard the following diagnosis during an ultrasound: "An internal birth defect: anencephaly." As in my case (bilateral multicystic dysplastic kidney), anencephaly is a fatal defect, that is, a baby can't live with it, she dies either at birth or soon after. It's the full or partial lack of the hemispheres of the brain, bones of the vault of the skull, and soft tissue, the result of abnormalities in the formation of the neural tube.

But in contrast to me, Zhanna found the courage in herself to walk her path to the end, moreover, in Russia. She carried the pregnancy to term and gave birth to her son Yegor at home; he died at birth.

April 2016. I meet Zhanna at the Anderson children's café. A delicate, short, uncertain girl with slender arms and a giant belly: she's pregnant again.[1] Zhanna arrives with her husband and six-year-old daughter. She deliberates for a long time, very seriously, about which table would be best for us to sit at so that she can see her husband and daughter in the play room, and they can see her. Then, she studies the menu just as seriously while choosing the correct tea. She clarifies the purpose for which I'm writing my book one more time. She certainly doesn't look like a person made of iron, capable of throwing down a challenge to the system.

Nonetheless, that's exactly what she did.

How did you decide to give birth at home with such a diagnosis? Wasn't it scary? That's some risk.

At first, it was very scary—while we didn't have all the information. The doctors were saying that if I gave birth in the hospital, it could only be by caesarian section. That no one would allow me to give birth on my own. In general, they said that giving birth to such a baby would be synonymous with death. That I had to think about my older child. That carrying a pregnancy to term with this kind of defect had never been done, it was

---

[1] As this book was going to press, Zhanna gave birth to a healthy son.

unknown how things would develop, the baby would die in the uterus, in general, everyone would die. From the moment of the diagnosis, in approximately the seventeenth week of gestation, all the doctors insisted that there was no choice.

Where and how was the diagnosis made?

First in the district clinic, later in the specialized Kulakov Center on Oparin Street. At the district clinic, first the doctor looked my ultrasound in silence, then she said: "Go take a walk in the corridor, I need the baby to turn over, and then I'll look again." When I returned, she was no longer alone but with a colleague. They both stood examining me, silently. I kept asking: "Is something wrong? Why are there two of you? Why aren't you answering me?" Finally, they said: "There's a serious pathology, anencephaly. There's one-hundred-percent evidence for termination." I asked: "And what if I don't terminate?" The doctor was surprised: "Why do you need this? Do you want me to show you pictures of children with these deformities, right now?" A doctor says this, without ceremony, to a woman who's just heard that kind of diagnosis! I answered: "No, thank you." Her idea was to immediately frighten me to such a degree that I wouldn't even think about prolonging the pregnancy. And the colleague whom she'd called said: "Even Down's children live at least somehow, but yours will lie there like a vegetable as long as he lives."

Did those words traumatize you—or, given the scale of the catastrophe, did the words even matter, compared to the diagnosis?

My husband and I even talked about it later. As a matter of fact, that turned out to be practically the most painful moment in our story—namely, the way they communicated the news to us. Without any tact or sympathy. With the proposal to show me other children with physical deformities, a minute after I found out that my baby would die. And even more how, just as soon as they see something's wrong, they begin to say "fetus with anomalies" and not "baby." Somewhere in the comments in online chat rooms, I read that in our country, it appears, this is the way medical people build a "healthy nation." By insistently arguing for a woman to abort if the baby has a pathology. After all, this way child mortality at birth is immediately reduced, and only healthy babies are born. It seems to me that this kind of agitation for termination is really about statistics.

What happened after that?

At the Kulakov Center on Oparin Street, they confirmed the diagnosis. Some old guy did my ultrasound. And as soon as he saw the defect, he completely stopped behaving the way people usually behave with pregnant women. Usually, they guide the sensor neatly over the stomach, talk about something. But he began to press down with all his might so that he could look at something better, to literally shake my stomach, to knock on it with the sensor—so that the baby would turn over, and it would be easier for him to see. Then, he called two other fellows, and they all looked together, talking among themselves: "Well, do you see it?" "Yes, it's all there. No other possibility. One hundred percent. Write the referral for termination." Among themselves! As if I weren't even there. They were talking about other possibilities, as far as I understood, because there's another, different defect that outwardly looks slightly similar to this one, where the brain is very deeply affected, and the baby is born severely disabled—but it's not fatal, that disabled child can live.

And what would you have done in that situation? If they'd told you that he'd live, but be severely disabled?

At that moment, most likely, I wouldn't have chosen to terminate the pregnancy. But they told me that mine wouldn't live. They said: "Come back by nine tomorrow, and be ready to terminate it."[2] And they added: "Don't give it a thought, there's nothing to think about." But I understood that I wouldn't be going anywhere at nine tomorrow. First, I needed to gather my thoughts, to find information about these kinds of cases. I went online— but I really didn't find anything about cases in Russia when people carried a pregnancy with anencephaly to term. There are many cases in which a similar diagnosis was made—but always afterwards: "I terminated the pregnancy." And I was searching for how such a pregnancy progresses, how the birth goes. In principle, I wanted to carry the pregnancy to term, but not at any price. I wasn't prepared to die and leave my husband a widower, my daughter an orphan. It just seemed strange to me that carrying such a pregnancy to term was supposedly impossible.

What did your parents say?

---

[2] It's now possible to terminate a pregnancy in the later stages at the Kulakov Center; in 2012, I was refused such a termination there.

They immediately said, of course, that it was necessary to terminate.

And your husband?

My husband wasn't sure. The main question was whether the choice really came down to pregnancy or the grave. In this situation, he wasn't prepared to take unnecessary risks. He said his main fear was losing me.

But wasn't there actually a risk of just that happening? That because of the non-standard size of the baby's head, something might go wrong during birth?

My contractions lasted six hours because of the size of the baby's head.

In fact, that period is usually measured in minutes.

Yes. A very small head, a deformed skull. Usually, the large head pushes through and opens the way, then everything else drops out easily. And here, we had a small head. That is, the head came out, but the shoulders were very wide in comparison with it—and they got stuck.

And all this happened at home?

Yes.

Was there any kind of back-up plan? If something went wrong—an ambulance and the hospital?

Yes, we thought about that possibility, but only in the most extreme instance: if we understood that we couldn't manage by ourselves. Because if we'd called an ambulance, this is what would've happened: either a caesarian section, meaning I wouldn't have been allowed to try to give birth on my own, or if the baby were already in the process of birth and dead, he'd have been dismembered. That is, maybe they were just trying to frighten me, but the doctors told me: well, they'll simply extract him in pieces, no one's going to stand on ceremony. And in any event, they'd have taken him away from me immediately. And not allowed us to say goodbye. Doctors think it's better for a woman not to see her dead baby. Besides, if the baby had been born in a maternity hospital by caesarian, there's a great probability that he'd have lived for a little while. They'd have taken him away and tried to "save" him, although there was no point in that, hooked him up to machines to be resuscitated—and they wouldn't have let me be there. I resolved, firmly: it's better for him to live just a minute, but be with me all of that minute, than an hour or a day on a machine, without me.

Was there any medical professional with you at the birth?

No, just my husband and a doula.[3] She has experience attending births, but not a medical education.

Why didn't you ask someone, even a midwife?

We wanted to ask a midwife, and we looked for one. We met several times with midwives. But they all refused. That is, no, at first, we simply looked for a maternity hospital in which we could give birth by private, paid contract. I was given various contacts, I phoned doctors, including some recommended to me by acquaintances. They refused. One doctor recommended by an acquaintance said: "You have to understand, no maternity hospital is going to take you because no one wants to spoil their statistics on child mortality." When we understood that it was going to be impossible to make arrangements with a good maternity hospital, we started looking for a midwife. We went to a meeting with midwives who were very highly recommended to us. As we drove, I rejoiced, thinking, they'll come to the birth, they'll help, and it'll be calmer for my husband and me. But they heard us out and refused. They said it was very dangerous, and we'd all die. We left— and my husband said: "Well, enough. We won't give birth at home." After that, I started looking for experience abroad. I discovered an English-language site devoted solely to this diagnosis. Through a translator, we wrote to the creators of that site. And in answer, they sent us statistics, descriptions, how births take place with this kind of diagnosis. They'd never had any cases of maternal death at all!

And you didn't have the idea to leave and give birth outside the country?

No. It just didn't occur to us.

Was it difficult psychologically to carry a doomed baby?

---

[3] A doula is an assistant who provides psychological, informational, and simple support at a birth; she can't administer medications.

It went up and down. Sometimes, I wanted the birth to take place early so that it would all be over. On the other hand, at some moments I didn't want the birth to happen because I understood that while he was inside, he'd be alive, but that after the birth, he'd go away. That kind of wavering went on all the time—but I didn't once regret deciding to keep the baby until the end. Although my relatives proposed numerous possibilities, doctors they knew, etc., who'd help me terminate everything quickly and forget. The main idea, for some reason, was that one needs to forget everything, as quick as can be. And I didn't want to forget.

I'm looking at you here—you certainly don't look like the Terminator, who's prepared to stand alone against everyone else. Where did you get the strength to oppose the system, to endure that pressure?

At first, it really did seem as if literally everyone was against me. But at some point, I simply decided it was my business and not theirs.

And was there any kind of hope for a miracle? That the baby would somehow survive?

No, there was no hope, no belief in magic, either. Purely theoretically, I knew that the baby might live, for example, for a few days.

And how was your daughter? She saw your belly, she probably asked questions?

Of course, she saw. But we told her immediately, look, you're going to have a brother, but you won't be able to play with him because as soon as he's born, he'll turn into a precious angel and fly to heaven. And during the birth, my parents took her.

She wasn't surprised by that explanation about angels? She took it in stride?

Well, she was four years old. It wasn't that surprising. But she asked: "Why is it that children born to other people don't turn into precious angels and fly away?" I told her that it varies. Our baby decided to become a precious angel. That's why he couldn't stay here with us at home, unfortunately. But all the same, in some way he'd always be with us. At four years old, she took that kind of information in stride, yes.

Someone treated you during your pregnancy?

For the better part of the pregnancy, I just didn't go to the doctors at the polyclinic, as I knew exactly what they'd say to me there. Only towards the end did I find a doctor-gynecologist who agreed to treat me privately, in spite of my diagnosis. Well, just so that someone made sure that everything was fine with my body.

How did your husband behave during the birth? Many people have assured me that a man isn't able to bear that kind of thing.

Initially, my husband thought that, most likely, he wouldn't be able psychologically to take that baby in his arms, to hold him. But when the birth happened, he took him. And later, he told me that he was very glad he actually did it. He said: "At that moment, I understood that my son had been born. I took him in my arms, spoke with him a little, and said goodbye." It was very important for him.

Did you receive any kind of psychological help after the birth?

No, there were no psychologists. But I observed a birth closure ritual.

What's that?

I did it with Natasha, the doula. Body wrapping after the birth. Specific points on my body were bound, with the help of scarves. On the whole, it's like re-living the birth. Voicing some of the fears. Everything is being remembered anew. And with this—with massage, a bath—the body is steamed, freed from fear.

You mean some kind of mystical ritual? Or does it have a purely physiological significance, as well?

I wouldn't say it's purely mystical. It's more as if, with the help of massage and the bath with herbs, they help the body open itself up.

Why exactly did Natalya, the doula, attend your birth?

When I got pregnant, I immediately agreed with her that she'd accompany me during the birth. Later, when they gave me the diagnosis, I wrote her that the situation had changed—and she turned out to be the only person who was prepared to stick with me until the end.

Didn't the medical danger in itself worry her?

She immediately began writing to her foreign colleagues and midwives—and they answered her that they had experience with such births and hadn't had a single fatality.

How pregnant are you now?

Thirty-five weeks.

Was it scary to be pregnant again?

Yes, very scary.

How did you live, at the end of that pregnancy? If we compare it, for example, with this trouble-free one? It seemed to me at the time that if I decided to carry the baby to term, that whole pregnancy, all of life would take place as if in the middle of some kind of dreary, black cloud...

No, there was no black cloud. The pregnancy lasted a long time—forty-three weeks. On the whole, I lived normally. Met with people, passed the time with them.

And when acquaintances saw your belly and congratulated you?

At first, when they congratulated me, I started to explain things. And then, I stopped explaining and just said: "Thank you."

Probably, you have a very strong nervous system? You're a very calm person.

Not at all. I'm very nervous, anxious. I just acted that way in order to be less nervous. It was simpler for me.

And besides the body wrapping, did you do anything else after the birth? A support group, perhaps?

No, no support groups. But over the course of forty days after the birth and death of the baby, I wore mourning. The way it was done earlier in our Slavic culture and tradition. For me, this was very important, psychologically. I made a special study of this question—what our ancestors did when a baby died. I prepared everything in advance: I bought black clothes, I didn't have any in my wardrobe, I don't like the color black in general, and it doesn't suit me. At home and on the street, I wore only black. Mourning extended to all spheres of life in general, not just clothes. No entertainment, no meetings with friends—none of that should happen for forty days. At home, all the mirrors were covered for forty days, a candle burned. As a matter of fact, if you enter fully into the condition of mourning, it's good psychological support. I tried to cry every day...

Tried? Meaning you didn't always want to?

The first days, of course, I wanted to. But with time, I had to specially make myself. As a matter of fact, if you allow yourself to weep, you can cry yourself out fairly quickly... In general, the idea is not to avoid your grief, not to pretend that nothing's happened, if you want to cry, cry, all of that helps. I also looked at casts of his little hands and feet. We made casts—they sell that kind of soft clay in the store, we bought it early, on purpose. Now we keep those casts. I also keep the pregnancy test. I also bought and keep a little baby bottle—as if it were his little bottle. And a onesie from a set—I bought one for the funeral, and there was one left over. It's a kind of material memory.

Keeping a material memory—was that your idea?

No, I just read about it on that English-language site. They wrote all about casts and other things there. About how people make a supreme effort to preserve that moment, because it's the only material memory that remains.

How did your daughter react to the practice of mourning?

Calmly. Sometimes, she asked questions. For example: "Why is that candle burning?" We answered her that it was for her brother, the precious angel, so he could see that we were thinking of him.

Did your husband also observe mourning?

No, he didn't wear mourning but, traditionally, men didn't wear mourning. Traditionally, a woman grieved both for herself and for the man. With regard to me wearing mourning—it was hard for him, of course, to look at a person who was always in black, and so forth. But later, he again came to the conclusion that I'd done everything right. After mourning, no unhealed, open wound remained. I knew that everything had happened, I'd seen my dead son, held him in my arms, and now I was fully immersed in my grief. And everything around me, the clothes, the mirror, told me that my grief surrounded me. Mourning surprised a few relatives, they didn't like the idea at all. They didn't understand why I "tortured" myself that way for forty days when it was necessary to simply "forget everything as quickly as possible," as if it had never been.

Who looked after your child while you were in mourning?

Traditionally, it's assumed during mourning that a woman is practically released from parental responsibilities. But that tradition presupposes a big house, in which several generations live, and that there are many other women who look after the children of the woman in mourning. They tried not to distract the woman from mourning—but also not to immerse the children in it. Naturally, it wasn't possible for us to do that. But my husband helped a great deal, my mama also helped. Naturally, my daughter was right here in the apartment all the time anyway, it was necessary to talk to her and sometimes join in some games. But with time, I learned how to switch between the two. It's simply an adjustment to our era.

And how did people look at you on the street? You went out on the street entirely in black?

Yes. It was summer, and I wore a black skirt, a black cardigan, and a black jacket when it was cold, bought especially for mourning. They looked at me normally. Later, on the fortieth day, we traveled to the grave, returned, took off all the covers from the mirrors, I took off my black clothes and put on other ones, pretty ones. And I felt that transition very keenly. Like a return into life. Like a return to life.

DEPUTY HEAD DOCTOR

for Obstetrics and Gynecological Care (Moscow)

"Only with permission and by order"

Query to Infectious Diseases Clinical Hospital No. 2
(Sokolinaya Gora)

Good day!

My name is Anna Starobinets, I'm a writer and journalist. At present, I'm finishing work on a book based on my personal experience and dedicated to the loss of a baby/late termination of pregnancy for medical reasons (fetal pathology, intrauterine fetal demise, etc.). The book will be published by Corpus. The first part of the text is autobiographical. The second part is interviews with women who have had similar experiences and also with German and Russian psychologists and doctors. Insofar as the maternity hospital that's part of Infectious Diseases Clinical Hospital No. 2 is, in fact, the leading establishment in which late termination of pregnancy for medical reasons takes place, I'd very much like to include discussion of this subject with specialists from the maternity hospital in the text. I'd be grateful for assistance in organizing an interview with the Deputy Head Doctor for Obstetrics and Gynecological Care, Yelena Viktorovna Lyalina, or with another doctor at the maternity hospital who performs termination of pregnancy and is prepared to speak with me on this subject.

The subject is difficult, painful, but important for many women, and it's important to society. Therefore, I very much hope for your cooperation and response.

My cell phone number is....

My email is....

Respectfully,

Anna Starobinets

03 80

Reply from Infectious Diseases Clinical Hospital No. 2

Good day.

All interviews with medical personnel take place only with permission and by order of the Moscow Department of Health.

Respectfully,

Ye. V. Lyalina

ଘ ଥ

I was unable to obtain responses to phone calls and letters from the Department of Health; my query also remained unanswered by the V. I. Kulakov Research Center for Obstetrics, Gynecology, and Perinatology on Oparin Street.

PATIENT NO. 2

Nastya, mama of Lada and Miroslav (Klin)

"Hello, my children are dead, can you talk to me about that"

In October of 2015, twenty-nine-year-old Nastya lost twins, a boy and a girl, at eighteen weeks of pregnancy. According to the doctors, by the time the ambulance delivered her to the hospital, it was already impossible to stop a miscarriage. However, for Nastya—a staunch opponent of abortion in any form, at any stage of pregnancy—it was very clear that her pregnancy, if it really was fated to terminate, would terminate by natural means, without medical interference. She didn't meet any understanding among the doctors and, literally risking her life, she went home, where the birth took place.

After a couple of months, Natsya tried to find a support group for parents who've lost babies, but she discovered that those kinds of groups don't exist in Moscow. Then, she organized one herself. Now, meetings take place regularly for Muscovites, and residents of other cities will soon be able to take part in those meetings by Skype.

Here, probably, it's important to underscore that the meetings are organized not by medical professionals or psychologists (as they are in Germany), but personally, by an interested "amateur." I attended one such meeting. In my view, it's very useful and, clearly, has a therapeutic effect. In this case, the "amateur" format is better than nothing at all.

Tell me, why did you end up in the hospital, and what happened there?

I'd had IVF, for physiological reasons, it's the only way for me to get pregnant.[1] Two embryos had implanted. But at the stage of eighteen weeks, there was a prolapse of the amniotic sac in the vagina. At the insistence of the midwife, we went to the hospital. But there, the doctors said that nothing could be

---

[1] In vitro fertilization.

done. Then I wanted to leave that hospital! Or go to a different hospital. We tried to find a hospital where they'd take us, but they all refused, including the Kulakov Center. No one wanted to spoil their statistics.

But in the hospital where you were, the medical personnel tried to somehow stop the process?

Yes, they gave me magnesia in an IV drip, papaverine, No-Spa. But really, what could they do? Nothing. I spent several days there on bed rest, and every day, several times a day, they came in and said: "Have an abortion, have an abortion, have an abortion."

Why weren't they prepared to wait for a spontaneous abortion, if there was really no chance?

They said it was impossible because then, I'd die.

From what?

From the fact that I'd supposedly developed sepsis. At first, they said that sepsis was beginning. And then, they started saying it had already begun.

Why "supposedly"? Did you have a high temperature?

Yes, towards the end, my temperature began to climb. But as soon as I got away from there, my temperature came down, immediately. I think it spiked because of nerves. They also said to me that if I didn't have an abortion, but gave birth myself, I'd start to hemorrhage. And that even if I didn't die, I'd lose my uterus. It was extremely strong pressure, they insisted that I have an abortion.

Did they let your husband in?

They let my husband in.

Where did all this happen?

In the city hospital, in Klin. I'm outraged at the behavior of the doctors. I think that a doctor may advise, may insist on some things, may even assign blame. But he may not openly oppose, may not forbid someone to leave the hospital. I had the feeling that I was in jail.

How did they forbid it?

Well, this is how. I said I wanted to go home. They said: "No, we won't let you." My husband said: "That's it, I'll take her, give me a wheelchair, please." They said: "No, we won't give you one." "Fine, I'll carry her in my arms." "No, we're standing here in the passageway and won't let you leave." That's insane! And then, they called a police detail.

And what did the police do?

They came, stood to the side—and that's it. They wrote: "Public order was not disturbed."

How did you manage to get out of there?

After the police left, two lawyers arrived. I wrote that I'd been warned I'd lose my uterus, I'd die, and so forth, if I left the hospital. Then they said to me: "It's somewhat illegible. Come on, now, read it aloud." I read it aloud, and they recorded me on a tape recorder. After that, they gave me a wheelchair, and we left. I have the transcript from the hospital.

She sends me a scan of the transcript by email. It lays out about the same story that Nastya told me, but with slightly different emphases:

> ... *Taking into account the worsening condition of the pregnant woman, the development of endometritis, the lack of prospect for the progression of the given pregnancy, termination of the pregnancy is offered to the patient, supplemented by antibacterial and infusion therapy. The patient and her husband categorically refuse the termination of pregnancy, insist on the transfer of the patient to the Kulakov Research Center for Obstetrics, Gynecology, and Perinatology.... The necessity for hospital care, and also the lack of prospect and the danger of further prolonging the pregnancy, and the irreversible consequences for the life and the health of the pregnant woman are explained to the patient and her husband in an easily understandable form.... Hospital lawyers are called for the legal preparation of the refusal of hospitalization.... A police patrol was called. In the presence of the district police captain [full name] and the senior police officer [full name], the condition of his wife is explained to Mr. [full name of Nastya's husband], and also the consequences of refusing the proposed treatment (antibacterial therapy, infusion therapy, termination of the pregnancy). Informed refusal of hospital care is prepared in the presence of lawyers for the Klin City Hospital. The patient is discharged from the department.*

The word "sepsis" is not in the transcript, but the phrase "incipient infected miscarriage" is there.

Leaving the hospital, you risked a great deal.

At that moment, I sincerely believed the doctors that I had sepsis. I realized that the outcome might be fatal. But I wasn't going to kill my children with an abortion, even if I died myself. They had to live their allotted time.

It seems to me, in that situation, when the children are doomed in any case, to give up your life—that's just a form of suicide. It's another thing entirely that the doctors, in theory, should have respectfully accepted your rejection of abortion and allowed the birth to take place a natural way, without stimulation. But that was a slippery moment with sepsis. If sepsis had really begun, according to their opinion, they were obliged to save your life.

No. If a person is conscious and in her right mind, she can refuse medical interference at any stage.

Did you have hope that the children would survive?

Of course.

What happened at home?

We arrived at night, everything was fine, my temperature fell. And the birth began in the morning.

Were any medical personnel present at the birth?

Yes, the midwife came, the one I'd gone to in preparing for the birth and with whom I'd planned to give birth. She examined me, said everything had come out, sat with me a little while to be certain that there was no hemorrhage. She made me eat. Then, she left, and she advised me to call an ambulance and the police. I think we might not have had to do that: as far as I know, in this country embryos become people only at twenty-two weeks. But we called. A conflict also arose with the ambulance, as I didn't want to go with them for cleaning out, and they insisted on it. I was already tired of all this pointless medical interference. And then the ambulance doctor said "This material must be taken for disposal" about our children. My husband answered: "I'll take *you* for disposal!" The ambulance doctor was extremely frightened and called the police. She told the police that my husband beat me and that we'd caused the abortion. The police tried to take my husband to the slammer, and the ambulance tried to take me to the hospital.

But they didn't?

In that situation, I turned out to have the clearest head, and I called a lawyer who specializes in family affairs. She talked on the speaker phone with the policeman and with the ambulance people, she said that they were breaking such-and-such laws and regulations. Was the person conscious? Conscious. That meant she could make her own decision about hospitalization. That was the end of things. Later, we ourselves buried the children. You can't legally bury children born at that stage. They aren't considered people. They're considered Class B biological waste. And if it had happened in the hospital, they wouldn't have given them to us. Because they were potentially dangerous. They were "not human," meaning it was forbidden to bury them in the cemetery. And burying them that way—there could be soil contamination, for example. And when I later went to a doctor recommended by an acquaintance for an ultrasound to see whether anything remained in my uterus, the first thing she asked me was "Did you bury them well? I'm not going to be named a co-conspirator later?"

That was the reason you didn't want to remain in the hospital? So that you could bury them?

For my husband and me, these children are absolutely the same kind of people as we are, as are other members of our family. We don't consider them some kind of future children. They're already children. How is it possible to leave children in the hospital for disposal? Besides, no one in the hospital would've given me three hours to give birth on my own. They absolutely would have interfered in the process. Then, they'd have given me a mandatory cleaning out. In general, I think it's best of all for a person to be born and die at home, surrounded by family. And since it turned out that my children were going to die, I wanted to at least have the chance to say goodbye to them. And I'm happy that we did everything exactly that way. It warms my heart that they didn't suffer. That they weren't torn into pieces. That they died peacefully.

... We're talking by Skype. I'm in Jūrmala, Latvia, and Nastya's in the Russian city of Klin. Through the computer screen, through interference, through cities and countries, she smiles when she says these words. It really does warm her heart that she said goodbye to her children. And that they departed in peace.

Here, it's possible to argue a great deal about whose side truth is on. About how normal or abnormal it is to be an ardent opponent of abortion. About what motivated the doctors trying to keep her in the hospital: was it an attempt to protect themselves from hypothetical problems, or to protect the patient from hypothetical complications, was it the instinct to "forbid, don't allow," or the precept to "do no harm." But there's no sense in having this fight, because it's beside the point.

It's entirely probable that, from the point of view of medical protocol, the doctors were right. That in this case, the gold standard of care is "termination of pregnancy supplemented by antibacterial and infusion therapy." However, from the human point of view, they did harm. They inflicted serious psychological trauma on Nastya and her husband. Because besides medical protocol, ethical protocol is also needed in this case. It's impossible and dishonest to demand sincere, human sympathy from all the doctors in the city of Klin towards every stubborn woman who doesn't want to obey an explanation "offered in an easily understandable form." In this case, a simple and clear plan of action, that same "ethical protocol," would have stood in quite well for sincere compassion: how should one behave with a patient who for a religious or any other consideration is not prepared to terminate a pregnancy, even at the risk of death? How should one behave if the patient doesn't trust you (and let's say that you're telling the truth—although the story about sepsis is somewhat murky)? If she hopes for a good outcome, if her reaction to terrible news is denial?

Unfortunately, no such protocol exists in the city of Klin or anywhere else in Russia. That's why every single doctor in every single situation behaves simply "on the whim of the moment." And instead of calling a psychologist for the patient, they call the cops. Instead of offering the patient a "second opinion" (that is, a doctor from another clinic who would have confirmed "the lack of prospect and the danger of further prolonging the pregnancy"), they throw themselves heroically across the opening, stand in doorways blocking the way out. And instead of expressing sympathy with the mother who's just lost her children, they express concern about the issue of "disposal of biological waste"...

The children were born dead?

They lived about twenty minutes. They stirred, opened their little mouths but, naturally, didn't breathe. While the placentas pulsed, they lived. And then, they quietly fell asleep.

What happened after that?

It seemed to me that I'd been skinned alive. At night, I had heart palpitations, I even underwent an EKG, but they didn't find anything. Later, I understood that these were panic attacks.

Did you look for psychological support?

I looked for a support group for women like me, but I didn't find any. The Gift of Life Fund sometimes organizes those kinds of meetings, but there was nothing in the near term. In the end, I was even glad that I didn't end up there. Later, people told me that there was a huge crowd, four hundred people. That is, a large-scale event, it would have been difficult for me there, and I'd have been disappointed. For our meetings, I understood that ten people was the absolute maximum, so that everyone can have the chance to speak and listen to others. If a person needs to speak, you can't cut them off. Because for many people, this is simply the only chance to talk about their lost children and be heard. Because for some reason, we who've lost unborn children are perceived in society as if we hadn't lost anyone.

How did you get the idea to organize support groups yourself?

At that time, I was a member of the Facebook group Open Heart, and I saw an invitation to a similar meeting in Petersburg.[2] I wrote: "We don't have that kind of thing in Moscow." And they answered me: "So, organize one." I asked: "How?" And they explained that the first thing to do was to find a meeting space. I found one. I wrote about the meeting on social media, through Vkontakte. Seven people came to the first meeting, that seemed very few to me. But when twelve people came to the next meeting, I understood that that was the limit. In my experience, the maximum length of the meeting must be not more than four hours—that should suffice for all the stories, the pouring out of emotion, the responses to the stories of others. If it's longer, it's too hard. Now, we're organizing Skype conferences for women who don't have the opportunity to come to a meeting in person. So far, there's been only a trial meeting by Skype—but everyone liked it. Of course, there are a few technical problems that affect the quality of these meetings. For example, a person is talking about her grief, and at the same time someone hears interference, or a cell phone chirps next to the microphone. But on the other hand, there are pluses, for example, if it becomes difficult for you, you can simply turn off the camera and sit listening and crying so that no one can see you.

---

[2] Open Heart is a closed group for women who've lost children.

And the fact that you're at home, you don't have to go anywhere, go out on the street—that is, indeed, an additional comfort.

According to the women at the meetings, what traumatized them most of all—aside from the loss of a baby, of course? Is there any kind of recurring traumatic experience connected to this sorrow?

The attitude of the medical personnel—that's the most painful point for almost all of them. That they were treated inappropriately. In general, I've never yet heard a story in which medical personnel behaved appropriately.[3] The second trauma almost all of them have experienced is the understanding that, even though "family is your support," "those dear to you will help in grief"—that's all a fairy tale. In reality, everything looks different. Those close to you give you to understand: go grieve somewhere else. For example, close relatives say, "Why are you crying? Enough crying, you have to keep on living!" No one wants to dirty their hands with you, your grief, and your condition. I myself ran into this. The majority of girls who come to us don't receive enough support from the family.

What did you run into?

I even stopped speaking to one of my close relatives because of this. She said the kind of things to me that wound me to this day. That this isn't the worst thing that can happen in life. That these children were given to me as a lesson, so I'd learn to love. I'd never have agreed to that kind of lesson of my own free will! I don't need that kind of lesson! I'd never have chosen "to learn to love" at the price of my children's lives. It would be better to stay ignorant, incapable, unloving, whatever you like—if only they'd lived. Another female relative argued that I couldn't say "I lost a baby"—"What's wrong with you, it wasn't a baby, it was an embryo." Those are such Soviet ideas—that the embryo is some kind of tadpole or baby turtle almost up to the ninth month.

What would have helped you, what kind of words? What would have made you feel better?

Compassion. There aren't any specially prepared phrases that can help. It helps if a person is prepared to share your pain and take a part of it on herself. But this is very difficult psychological work, and not everyone's able to

---

[3] At the meeting I attended, practically all the women complained of the callousness of the doctors or of being pressured by them.

do it. You have to have a very brave heart to be able to share the pain of a person whose whole life at a given moment consists of pain. If you understand that you don't have enough sincerity or strength to do that, then it's better not to say anything at all. You can just be silent and stay close. Or think about how you can help. In any case, it has to be from the perspective of "I'm here," rather than "I'm looking down." That is, I'm not going to teach you now why all this happened to you, or that all this is nonsense and "That's enough, pull yourself together" or "You think you're the only one?" For example, I went to church, told the priest what had happened to me. And he answered me: "Well, so what? You're not the only one." What kind of answer is that? My grief doesn't lessen because the children of many other people die. For him, this was ordinary natural selection. Well, yes, natural selection, I won't argue. Weak females like me can't carry descendants to term. Nature is very cruel. That should console me? So, if even the priest can't find words—what should I expect of ordinary people? Really, a priest should be like a psychologist, only better.

Are you a religious believer?

I'm a believer, but not completely observant. I have my own ideas about God. For example, I confess, but I don't take communion. Because I don't like the idea of eating the body of Christ or drinking his blood. I'd like to interact with him in some other way.

And you didn't try to contact a psychologist?

A psychologist was recommended to me, but a visit to her cost three thousand rubles. We don't have that kind of money, we're trying hard to economize on everything. That is, for one visit, of course, it's possible to find such a sum. But what's really needed is a course of treatment, a minimum of ten sessions. I called the public psychological assistance service several times. I called—and hung up the phone. I have no idea how to start that conversation: "Hello, my children are dead, can you talk to me about that?"

Maternity Hospital Doctor

Christine Klapp, Doctor of Medicine, Head Doctor,
Charité-Virchow Obstetrical Clinic (Berlin)

"This is about fate, not about fault"

Frau Klapp came to work at Charité at the beginning of the 1990s—and over the course of a few years, she completely changed the clinic's approach to the late termination of pregnancy. In fact, she reformed the existing system—not just in the medical, but in the psychological sense. Frau Klapp considers the creation of a special "quiet room" in which parents may say goodbye to their children to be one of her most important accomplishments.

One of Christine Klapp's additional specializations is the mind-body connection in crisis situations. Besides gynecological consultations, she also conducts psychological consultations for women and couples at the clinic. She herself has lost two children, therefore, her experience isn't just professional, but human, personal. She's able to look at this grief from both sides—from both the inside and the outside.

What was the approach to late termination of pregnancy in Germany in the past?

Until the end of the 1970s, the termination of a pregnancy after twelve weeks wasn't generally possible. If a woman for some reason needed to do that, she went to the Netherlands. Later, the late termination of pregnancy was permitted in Germany for medical reasons, including psychiatric reasons. But the approach to such terminations didn't suit me. When I came to work at Charité in the beginning of the 1990s, we started an action committee made up of doctors, midwives, nurses, and a member of the clergy. The goal of the group was to help women cope psychologically with late termination and miscarriage and go through the grief process. We strove to make changes in the process. For example, we insisted that a woman had the right for someone close to her to be with her in the hospital—a partner, relative, or friend to stay with her overnight. And that it's generally the right thing to have both parents present at the termination.

Why is that the right thing?

When we began the practice of allowing a partner to be present in the 1990s, it very quickly became clear that it was better for both of them that way. It's well known that men and women experience this grief differently. When a man is present at the termination, he understands what happened much better, and it becomes their shared experience. Most men wouldn't choose to be present at the termination if their women didn't need them, but when they're there, they're usually quite emotionally involved. They say that they've felt a deep closeness to both their wife and their child. The presence of the partner helps prevent a future situation when the woman is still deeply burdened by grief but the man is already back to normal. It helps them stay together. If a man isn't involved in the process of the termination, he doesn't understand how to behave later. For example, he'll say to his woman: "Don't think about it. Forget it." And if the woman lights a candle in remembrance of her child, for example, he might say: "Don't do that, it's too much."

What other changes did you strive for?

Until the 1990s, those fetuses lost as a result of late abortion and miscarriage in East Germany were destroyed—for example, incinerated together with all the other medical waste after surgery. Here in West Germany, we'd already been burying them in the ground for several decades. There was a special place in the cemetery for such babies, but there wasn't any open, public burial ceremony. We strove to ensure that there'd be an official ceremony, with a member of the clergy. The kind of ceremony to which a woman might come, together with her family, and say goodbye to the baby. In 1995, we managed to do that. Now, Charité has two cemeteries for these kinds of babies: one in Wedding and another in Reinickendorf.

My baby is buried in Reinickendorf. Who pays for these cemeteries, for the funerals?

Charité.

Really? I thought that the church...

No. Charité takes on all the costs, including the arrangement of the graves and care for them, the flowers, and Charité also pays for the funeral ceremony. With regard to church officiants, we have clergy members of various confessions here at the clinic who are invited to the funeral with the parents, to comfort them, if need be. That was also s 1990s.

And before the 1990s, when there was no official funeral ceremony, could parents visit the graves of these babies? Did they know where to go?

In theory, they could have found out where the grave was and visited it. But at that time, no one among the medical personnel could have imagined that there existed parents who wanted to know where babies lost during pregnancy were buried. And most women didn't ask those questions. Perhaps they just didn't dare to ask. At the beginning of the 1990s, a number of terrible rumors about this were played up in the media. For example, that the bodies of these babies were used to pave roads. Of course, that was simply a fabrication, nothing of the sort ever took place, but in the absence of information, the imagination creates monsters. Not so long ago, I received a letter from the husband of a woman who lost her baby in the 1980s. She was so distraught and suffered so much after what happened that she never dared to get pregnant again. And now, after decades, she'd begged her husband to find out where that baby was. He turned to me—and I found his grave.

And how was the late termination procedure itself done at that time? Did they use anesthesia, for example?

Yes. But at the beginning, psychoactive sedatives were used, along with analgesics. We also changed that because women would say afterwards: "I don't remember anything! That was such a precious moment, the chance to say 'Goodbye' to my baby, to look at her—and now she's gone, and I don't even have any memory of her!" It took years to understand that for practically all women, it's better to see their dead baby. Many times, I've spoken with women who deeply regret that they didn't have the chance to see the baby. Later, they had terrible visions on that subject, they imagined their baby as a repulsive monster—especially in those cases where it was known that there was some kind of birth defect. Then, I thought: possibly, it would be better for them simply to see the real baby instead of what they imagined. I wasn't certain—I just assumed it. My colleagues and I turned to the Anglo-American experience, read the specialized literature in English. And all the facts showed that I was right—it's easier for women that way. Since that time, I've attended many mothers who've lost children late in pregnancy and agreed to look at the babies. Ninety-five percent were happy that they did.

What is the psychological mechanism? Why does this help, seeing your dead baby?

Because it allows you the chance to realize that the baby really exists and is really yours. It's not some kind of terrible vision or nightmare—it's your baby, although she's dead. And you're really her parent. And will always stay her parent. It's also a very good idea to give that baby a name. In Germany, by law, a baby is considered a person if her weight at birth is five hundred grams or more, or even if her weight is lower but she demonstrates signs of life after birth—breathing, a heartbeat. In this case, the parents are required to receive official documents for her—a certificate of birth (and death), of course, with a name. However, since 2013, they're not required, but have the right if they want to receive official documents about why she died, regardless of the length of the pregnancy or the baby's weight. They may also go and get these documents for babies they lost prior to 2013…

… After I returned to Moscow, I clarified that the Russian medical criteria for birth of a person in many ways correspond to German ones. However, the devil is in the details, as they say. According to Russian Federation law, twenty-two weeks of pregnancy and a newborn weight of five hundred grams are the criteria. If the length of pregnancy is less than twenty-two weeks or the weight is lower than five hundred grams, the baby will be considered a person only after he's shown the ability to survive more than seven days after birth. In all other cases, the baby remains "just a fetus." His parents can't receive official documents for him—birth or death certificates.

At that time, in the 1990s, we came to the conclusion that the majority of parents greatly value some kind of material memory of their baby. Therefore, at discharge, we always try to hand them a photo of the baby and a footprint. Sometimes, we also give parents little clothes, so they can dress their babies as they say goodbye. For example, we often use little sleeping sacs in order to bury babies, and small pieces of the fabric may be handed to the parents as a keepsake.

Do you insist that a woman must look at her baby?

No, of course not, it's wrong to insist, we can only recommend. I think that the doctor should say to the parents: "You may look at your baby, if you want to." The doctor should emphasize that this is fully possible. Because the majority of people up to this point are certain that it's either forbidden—or, if it's not forbidden, that it's a bad idea. I try to persuade them that it's necessary, first of all, to listen to their own feelings and make a decision in accordance with those feelings. If they aren't sure immediately after the birth whether they want to see the baby, I tell them: "You don't have to decide right now, you have time, we'll keep your baby here in the clinic for another two to three days." It took a very long time for the doctors to work out such an approach. At the beginning of the 1990s, many of my colleagues here at Charité were saying: "Ugh, that's not right, that's awful. The parents will have nightmares after they see that." But today, absolutely everyone is convinced that, yes, it's better for the parents if they're together in the clinic, and better if they see the baby and say goodbye.

... I listen to her and understand that, in our approach to the termination of pregnancy for medical reasons, Russia is two-and-a-half decades behind Germany. At a minimum. The situation that was considered the norm in Berlin in the 1980s is now considered the norm in Moscow, in 2016. And we haven't yet had reformers like Christine Klapp.

What can help a woman psychologically when termination at the clinic is already behind her? For me, for example, this was a period when I badly needed to talk about what had happened, but everyone around me operated under the idea that I needed to forget everything "as fast as possible."

First of all, the official funeral ceremony helps. Because it shows respect. Most women feel better if they see members of their family demonstrating respect for their grief and their loss. When a mother loses a baby who's a year or two old, for example, the whole family usually comes together around her, so as to comfort her. But when it's "just a fetus," relatives often say (and in earlier times, especially, loved to say): "Well, it wasn't yet a baby." Or: "You're still young, you'll still give birth to many normal children." But these kinds of words just make it worse. Because that baby—that baby was part of your life plan. You'd prepared to change your life for the next twenty years because of that baby! And now there's no more baby, and no more life plan, and without that plan, it seems to you that your life has ended. I myself lost a baby at nineteen weeks during my first pregnancy. That happened long before I came to work at the Charité clinic. And I lost a second child when he was eighteen years old. Therefore, I know very well what I'm talking about. Not just as a doctor—I have personal experience.

What I usually say to parents who've lost a child is: the period of grief will take some time. No one knows how long grief will last, but most likely all four seasons of the year will pass before it gets better.

Yes, that's how it was. All four seasons of the year.

Because that was your plan, you imagined all this: spring with the baby, summer with the baby, Christmas with the baby, and so on... Later, grief starts to overwhelm you from time to time, in waves. When you see someone with a baby, you feel sharp envy. A few parents cross to the other side of the street when they see a strange baby carriage. To a certain extent, this behavior's normal.

For a while, I really did avoid contact with young children, didn't meet with my friends who had babies. But I felt guilty. What's better, from the psychological point of view: to not torment yourself and avoid such contacts or, on the other hand, to master yourself and force yourself to admit that there are a vast number of living babies on the earth, and that you can't hide from all of them?

It's not a black-and-white situation. I think it's best of all to tell your friends something like this: "I can't see you right now, please understand. But don't be shy about calling and writing—I want to stay in touch. You can invite me to visit—but I'm not sure that I'll be able to accept. Please don't be offended if I decline." If you've already mustered up the courage to visit friends who have young children, you can say: "I want to see you, and perhaps everything will be fine. But it might also happen that after five minutes, I'll feel that I can't bear it. Then, I'll leave." Most of your friends will understand. By the way, they also feel very unsure. If you don't explain what you feel, they won't understand what they can talk about with you and what they can't, therefore they'll try to avoid certain subjects or simply avoid meeting you.

And what about interactions with the older generation?

Many women complain to me that their mothers say something like this to them: "It wasn't a baby, it was still unformed, it only seemed to you that you saw a real baby." Our parents are a different generation, they have a different mentality and a different education—they simply didn't learn these things. It's possible, for example, to show them a photo of the baby. Here, you can call a photographer who specializes in filming the so-called "star babies"—dead babies.

... She shows me photos of well-dressed dead babies. In pink and blue caps, in one-sies with bears, in baskets decorated with flowers. With closed eyes, with hurt, pursed lips. In colorful sleeping sacs—in which they'll sleep forever. In one of these photos, the mother's hand is visible—she's smoothing the cheek of her "star baby." I look at the photo and say, automatically, without thinking:

When I touched him, he was very cold.

He had to be cold. Just so that you could look at him. Otherwise, the pro-cess of change, the process of decay, begins very quickly. We have a special refrigerator with a fan for them here. In any case, even without the refrig-erator, the dead person would be room temperature. That's also not very pleasant. But a completely cold body is even more shocking. Therefore, if the parents don't want to see their baby right after birth, but the next day, we try to remove the baby from the refrigerator for an hour before that. And we try to prepare the parents for the fact that the baby changes very quickly, even in the refrigerator, he retreats further and further, every day he becomes more dead.

After this loss, how does a woman construct a relationship with her husband? After some amount of time, even a very understanding husband tires of constantly talking about a dead baby.

I suggest leaving grief a definite place in life, that is, setting aside a specific time frame for it. Most often, it goes this way: the woman is still thinking just about the baby she lost, and the man has already buried himself in work for a long time—in this grief, the man has left the woman many steps behind. In such a case, it makes sense to name a special day—for example, the date when the baby died, let's say the twelfth of every month, or every day, if necessary. And at a specific time, for example, at six in the evening, sit together with a glass of wine, or a lighted candle, or both. Maybe turn on music, hold hands, embrace, possibly don't even talk—simply think together about the baby you've lost. Half an hour, for example. It will be a half-hour of very concentrated thought and remembrance—and at the same time, closeness. On the man's part, it will not just be a tribute of respect for the baby—but also of respect for the woman's grief. Most men are fully capable of enduring these half-hours—if they know that it's really a half-hour. That this pain, this grief, has some kind of limit, that it won't be all-embracing and all-penetrating, won't fill up every corner of your home and your life. Yes, grief must have some limits, it's possible to compress it and give it some kind of shape. At first, possibly, you'll need to have these half-hours every day. But with time, less frequently: two times a week, once a week, once a month...

After a time, I began to have panic attacks.

That happens in these cases. Panic attacks, depression, or sleeplessness. A panic attack is usually a reaction to some kind of event, to an irritant, but sometimes it can happen without an irritant—or you simply may not see the irritant. It's a variant of post-traumatic stress syndrome, we find it in about 10 percent of women. Often, the panic attacks start at the time when the woman should have been giving birth, if she hadn't lost the pregnancy and the baby. Your body remembers the date, remembers what it was preparing for—and it feels something's wrong now, not according to plan, even if your conscious self doesn't take part in this. It's simply that your body had a perfect plan—the birth of a healthy baby at the right time. You gave birth to a dead baby at the wrong time, but it's as if the original plan were still being followed. It's the mind-body connection. Usually, this kind of mind-body manifestation passes with time. But you can try to help yourself without waiting for time to pass. For example, you can go to the cemetery where the baby is buried or if, for example, the cemetery's located in another city, you can go to church and light a candle for the baby. To remind yourself that the baby is real—and that she's dead. A second possibility is not to be alone when panic attacks take place. Call friends or relatives, spend time with them, talk. There are universal psychotherapeutic methods for treating post-traumatic stress syndrome—for example, imagining a hopeful place, a refuge for yourself, in which you'll be calm and things will be fine. But if post-traumatic stress syndrome is very strong and doesn't go away over a long period, then it's worth turning to a psychotherapist.

If there are older children in the family, is it better to tell them the truth about what happened?

Yes, it's better to tell the truth. Because otherwise, they think: "Oh, what have I done? I've probably done something terrible because Mama and Papa are so sad." Children under age eight can't understand what happened, but they feel that something happened and usually blame themselves for it. Or, they start to think that their parents don't love them anymore. Children a little older have enough imagination to understand what happened—and to imagine something very terrible. We recommend telling the truth but possibly not the whole truth. For example, it's not a good idea to communicate that you made some kind of choice and that you terminated the pregnancy. It's possible to simply say that the baby was very ill and didn't have a chance of surviving.

What about one's relationship with God in this situation? Including in the situation of this choice? In Russia, many women go to church and consult with the priest about whether to terminate a pregnancy or not. And the father gives advice according to his understanding of good and evil.

We also have that kind of problem here. For example, the Catholic church forbids abortion at any stage, for any reason. The majority of modern priests, so I hope, haven't lost their connection to reality and don't forbid women to terminate. But they can't officially permit it, and I can easily imagine a situation when a priest from a small town says to a woman: "No, the termination of a pregnancy is forbidden, it's a sin." In this sense, it's easier with the Protestant church. That's why we strive to partner with trustworthy clergy members, mainly Protestants. Frau Violet, with whom you spoke at Charité in 2012, is one of these, by the way. Our clergy members are closer to psychologists in the way they work. They offer support.

I had a constant feeling of guilt. That I was to blame for the formation of the mutations. That I took away my child's life. That I didn't pay enough attention to my older daughter because I was too consumed by grief.

The feeling of guilt is very typical and generally a normal reaction. The main thing is that it doesn't last too long and doesn't grow—in that case, a psychotherapist is needed, to work with the woman and her partner. It's very important to convey to the woman that it's not her fault—that these things just happen. This is about fate, not about fault.

If a woman becomes pregnant again, how does she deal with her fears? I had the feeling that everything was repeating, all over again.

Well, in the first place, it's necessary to do an ultrasound and all the necessary tests to satisfy oneself—objectively – that the situation isn't repeating itself. And subjectively, it's useful to concentrate on details and things that are unique to the new pregnancy, that distinguish it from the previous one. Different events take place. Maybe the baby moves a little differently inside. If that doesn't help, it means that the pregnant woman needs the supervision of a psychotherapist. Sometimes, the woman feels herself to be guilty before the baby she lost when she gets pregnant again. It's necessary to understand that, even if that baby isn't with you, all the same, he's a member of your family and your personal history and in that way, he'll always be with you. That this isn't the "substitution" of one baby for another. There's room for both. A few women don't want to get pregnant again at all because they're afraid they'll forget their dead baby then. But they'll never forget her. And sometimes we come to say something like this: "No, the dead baby won't be jealous of the living one and won't feel offended. If he's in heaven or somewhere else, he'll likely think: it's great to have a sister or brother!"

And if the pathology repeats anyway? Is it harder for women in that case than it was the time before?

On the one hand, yes, it's harder. But on the other hand, the woman knows that she's already survived emotionally and physically in this situation one time—and that means she'll survive again. And survival is hope. Hope for a different fate. Sometimes, I meet women whose babies had no birth defects at all, but for some reason they lose them, time after time, three or four months into the pregnancy. There are those to whom that's happened six times—and there isn't a single living baby. Sometimes they say: "That's it. I'm not ever going to try to have a baby again—I'm done." But I try to encourage a woman not to give up, even in that case. Yes, she knows what she's risking. But there's always the possibility that things will go well on the seventh try. I don't try to convince her of that, I say: "Just wait. Never say 'never.' It's possible that things will be different in a couple of years."

Do you have any kind of general rules about how to tell a pregnant woman about an unfavorable diagnosis?

We specifically train doctors and students in how to convey bad news. But there's a problem in that you arrive at the ultrasound in an excellent mood, you see your baby on the screen, you're happy, then you notice the doctor's face looks too serious, and she talks too little to you, not the way things normally are, and your heart goes cold... And then the doctor has to tell you this, no matter what. And everything changes radically for you in a second, and you aren't prepared for it. The right thing for a doctor to do in this case is to say something like this: "I'm so sorry, but I have bad news for you." And then, the news itself. There's no way to say it gently, or by degrees. You can only say it so it's clear; the doctor understands that it's very difficult for the woman to hear it. Then, the doctor can say: "Please, stay here as long as you want, have a cup of tea, you don't have to decide anything right now, if you want, we can call your husband or a friend to come and get you." Sometimes, the woman needs to come back for another consultation to grasp what happened, that is, it requires more than one visit to give her bad news. But in any case, a good, professional doctor must show the woman that he sympathizes with her. He doesn't have to cry together with her, but he has to show that he understands how difficult it is for her.

What does a woman do, having found out about the unfavorable diagnosis?

According to my personal statistics, when the fetus is discovered to have a lethal pathology, most women decide to terminate the pregnancy. But in the last two years, we've had a special palliative subunit here, and they encourage women in their intentions—or simply explain to women that it's possible—to carry the baby as long as possible, to carry the pregnancy to term and give birth the natural way. If the birth defect is lethal but the baby can live for a time, they offer palliative assistance so that the baby doesn't suffer from pain or hunger, but that requires the parents to understand that, in these cases, they won't undertake any life-prolonging therapy, such as dialysis, or a ventilator for the lungs. So, the women who decide to carry a pregnancy to term in these situations are a minority, but it's growing, bit by bit. They make this choice either because their religion doesn't allow them to do otherwise, or simply because they want to be next to their children as long as possible.

And if the pathology isn't lethal?

If it isn't lethal, but a serious pathology or even Trisomy-21 (Down's Syndrome), nine women out of ten decide to terminate the pregnancy because they aren't prepared to complicate their lives. But they must recognize that they're choosing this for themselves and not because of the baby. "Oh, my poor baby, it's better for you not to be born into this world than to suffer!"—that won't do. A woman doesn't have the right to decide whether a child's life is worth living. What she can decide is this: "It's too difficult for me and the members of my family to have a baby with this kind of health condition." By law, the word "difficult" here means a condition of the mind, the soul. And if a doctor gives a referral for termination of the pregnancy because of fetal pathology, he does so only if he agrees that the birth of that baby will damage the psyche of the mother. One doctor gives the referral for termination, but a different doctor must perform the termination. And every doctor has the right to refuse to do a termination for ethical considerations. For example, if it seems to her that the baby's problem is not sufficiently serious to take away that life. No one can compel us, doctors, to do that. If one refuses, the woman looks for another who'll agree. Because, by law, the woman decides for herself what's a big problem and what's not. I've come across a situation when a woman received a referral for termination because the baby had a cleft lip.[1] That pathology isn't lethal and generally isn't too serious. But that woman already had two children with cleft lips, they'd gone through many operations, her husband had left her—therefore, she received a referral for termination. But at the same time, by law, doctors had the right to refuse to do that termination for her. Until 1995, it was officially possible to make a decision about the termination of a pregnancy because of a birth defect with an argument such as "Oh, my poor baby, you don't need to suffer." But it's not ours to decide whether the baby should live or not. At the legal level, we ensured that the parent decides only for herself.

I heard that you've made a special room at Charité where mothers say goodbye to their babies.

Yes, together with my colleague, the midwife Frau Burst, we ensured that there's now a room at Charité for saying goodbye. It's also called the "quiet room." It's right here in the department. It was very important to us that it be located right here, in the maternity hospital, in the place where life begins, and not somewhere on another floor, or in the basement. And all the same, that it be set a little bit apart. So that it's possible to sit in quiet, but then open the door and find yourself among people, in the center of life, and find yourself part of that life and not alone underground. We turned to students at the Berlin School of Design and presented them with a practically impossible assignment. The sole space we had was a tiny room of just over sixty-four square feet, with two doors and no windows, that we'd been using to store medical instruments. And we asked them to turn that room into the kind of place where parents could say goodbye to their children. We told the students about the kind of grief a woman experiences and what happens to the babies. The young people (eighteen to nineteen years old) identified not only with the parents but with the children. They broke into groups of four and created model design projects, lighted and fully equipped. One group made a kind of jungle—their room was bright and green, a person would feel as if she were in a botanical garden. Another group created something absolutely hard and austere, they used mainly shades of grey, and they hung a cross on the wall. I said to them: "Think again about that cross. We also have other religions here in the clinic."

---

[1] A so-called "hare lip."

Their idea was that the space should be as austere as possible – so that nothing would distract from thoughts about the dead baby... In the end, they offered us six models. We liked a proposal by four girls, and we instructed them to create the room. They did everything themselves. They sewed everything made of fabric. They themselves went to Ikea for the furniture. There's a minimum of furniture, the room's very peaceful, the colors are mainly white and blue. There's a sofa and a place where you can place the basket with the baby. Also, there were four lamps in the form of globes that give off a gentle light. Now, there are just three. One of the lamps was stolen recently. Everything in the room, from design to construction, cost one thousand euros. We chipped in ourselves to collect that thousand... Would you like to see it? Our room for saying goodbye?

I would.

Midwife

Cornelia Burst, Senior Midwife, Maternity Department,
Charité-Virchow (Berlin)

"Living children can be born without me"

Cornelia Burst, a colleague and the main comrade-in-arms of Dr. Christine Klapp, has worked as a midwife since 1986 and at Charité since 1995. Then, in the mid-1990s, Klapp and Burst created the room for saying goodbye.

Now, Cornelia and I are sitting in that room—a tiny space without windows, outfitted in white and light-blue pastel colors. Cornelia explains that, according to psychologists, this spectrum of colors calms mothers who've lost their little babies. But in my case, the spectrum clearly doesn't work. I'm uncomfortable in this room. It's too cramped. Too stuffy. It looks too much like the room for saying goodbye in the other Charité building, a room created along the lines of, and similar to, this one. The room in which I myself said goodbye to my baby three years ago. Same sofa, same armchair, same little table, and same smell. The smell of faded flowers, scented candles, and death. I don't remember if there were windows in that other room. I don't remember if the same painting hung on the wall there as here: a lonely balloon floating in the endless sky. None of that's important. The single difference for me is that today, there's no basket with my dead child on this little table.

Frau Burst is a round, short-of-breath woman with a simple face and large hands. On the Charité website, she's listed simply as a midwife, without any further specialization. However, she has a specialty, and she chose it herself. She attends all births, but if anyone in the clinic is terminating a pregnancy in the later stages, or if someone has lost a fetus in utero or is beginning to miscarry late in the pregnancy, in a word, if a stillbirth is expected—they call Cornelia Burst.

It's probably difficult for you as a midwife to attend births that end with the death of the baby. Isn't the whole point of your profession to bring new life into the world?

Many people think that my job's unbearable, that it's continuous pain. For most midwives, stillbirth and the termination of pregnancy because of a serious pathology—that's really very difficult. For me, it's not. In such births, there's also a great deal of light. Usually, the midwives ask me to substitute for them. And I always agree to that work, I love it. I'm a "rock in the storm" for women at these kinds of births, I'm much more important for stillbirths than ordinary births, where healthy, living children are born. They can be born without me.

Do you remember the first time you attended this kind of birth?

Of course. When I was still a beginning midwife, in 1986, an acquaintance telephoned me. She said that a close friend who was pregnant had experienced a great misfortune—the embryo lacked half a heart (hypoplastic left heart syndrome) and wouldn't live past birth. That woman was under terrible stress and was frightened. She had to decide right away whether to terminate the pregnancy or carry it to term, give birth—and say goodbye. She had no hope that the baby would survive, it's a very serious defect, children who have it don't survive past three days. But she decided to carry it to term. And she asked me to attend the birth. I promised to try. It was a little frightening for me. I said: "Please, God, help me!"—and it turned out to be a wonderful experience. They gave her anesthesia, she was in no pain at all. The baby was born, on the outside he was entirely normal, beautiful—a real gift for that woman. They immediately laid him on her chest, no one took him away, and no one tried to "save" him. He lived a day and a half. And the first day of that day and a half was absolutely normal, he felt fine.

But how is it possible to interpret that day and a half, that day, as a "gift"? If you know for certain that he won't be with you later? Was this woman really not in tears and despair all that day and a half?

She was already prepared for what would happen. The only question was whether the baby would die during birth or would live for a little while afterwards. She knew all through the final months of the pregnancy. She said: "I don't plan to terminate anything, let nature decide." That was her inner feeling; it might be different for another woman. Of course, she didn't immediately come to the decision to carry the pregnancy to term. No one comes to that decision immediately. The first reaction is almost always "Take this away from me as quickly as possible!" It takes time to think through the situation and sort out your feelings. It's important not to pressure the woman, important that she has a choice... So, then, after that case, all my colleagues said to me: "Oh, poor Cornelia, how unlucky you were, how difficult for you to end up working with that birth, what a terrible experience." And I heard them and thought that, in fact, that wasn't how it was. It was the opposite, even. The atmosphere at that birth was amazing, as if some kind of extra, special light had been lit that filled the whole room. Her husband was at the birth. Everyone was very calm. No one fussed over the baby. They were given a separate room so that they could be there with the baby, although back then, in 1986, that still wasn't customary. And, yes, that woman perceived the birth of the baby and the day and a half of his life as a gift. She never regretted it afterwards. When you know that your baby won't live, the situation is terrible. But even in that terrible situation, there may be good, radiant, happy moments.

Happy moments?!

Yes. After that case, I got the impression that if a woman is in good hands, she might feel happiness, even in that kind of situation. They named that baby Carlo. Two years later, that mother gave birth to a healthy baby, I also attended that birth. But to this day, I remember Carlo with tenderness. There's a beautiful photo in which he's lying on her chest. He had a short life, but it was a life. For me, it was important in the experience with Carlo that I was able to help a woman bear the unbearable, to live through what might seem impossible to live through: to give birth to a baby and allow him to die on your chest... Of course, not all woman react that way if their children are doomed. Many times, I've attended births of completely "frozen," icy women who didn't want anything, not to look at their baby, not to touch her. That's what's really difficult for me—when a woman is "frozen." But it's my duty to accept that situation, too. A few ask us to do a caesarian section so that they don't participate in the process at all. Or they say: "Take away the baby as quickly as possible, as soon as she appears!"

That's exactly what I said. I was afraid to look at him. Afraid he'd be scary.

They aren't scary.

But there really are scary ones. With real, visible deformities.

If something is wrong, for example, with the head, you can put a cap on the baby. This is exactly the task for a midwife like me—to "present" the baby so that it isn't scary for the mother, so she can see, on the other hand, his beauty. For the tiniest babies, for example, I use the shell of an ostrich egg. I paint the shell, lay the baby in it, as if in a cradle, and show the mother.

Where do you get ostrich eggs?

Eggs? What do you mean, where? At an ostrich farm. There's one near Berlin. I sent them an email that I was a midwife at Charité and that I regularly need ostrich eggs...

Did you explain to them why you need the eggs?

Of course, I explained. That's exactly why they send them to me, free of charge.

If a woman doesn't want to look at her baby, in an ostrich shell or not, and asks you to "take her away as quickly as possible"—then do you take the baby away as quickly as possible?

Yes, but then I give the woman time and a chance to reconsider. There's always time left. Nothing has to be decided immediately—later, it's possible to regret things very much. The most important hours are the six to eight hours after birth, very often a woman needs that long to want to see the baby. Sometimes, it takes a little more time—for example, a day, although after twenty-four hours the baby already looks different, he's capable of changing a great deal. But all the same, we recommend looking at the baby. Because in any case, imagination is crueler than reality. In reality, the parents usually just see beauty. It's very important to see that this is your child, and that she's not a monster. "Oh, look, she has your lips and my nose!..." Once, I was walking somewhere along the street, I saw a billboard I liked a lot, and I took a picture of it. I love to photograph billboards... Here it is. See? "Everything you look at with love is beautiful."

She flips through the photos in her antediluvian cell phone: the faces of unknown people, posters with public service announcements, billboards, and tiny infant bodies in ostrich shells elaborately decorated with pink feathers flash past. Finally, she finds the right photo, with the slogan "Everything you look at with love is beautiful." She's strange, this Cornelia, photographing public service announcements on her phone. People say "not entirely of this world" about people like her.

And you... How do you look at these dead babies of strangers?

The same way I look at the living babies of strangers. I generally do exactly the same thing with them as I do with living babies. I wash them, dress them. I talk to them.

What do you talk about?...

I tell them: "Hello, welcome. How beautiful you are! How sad that your life was so short."

... In the cramped room for saying goodbye, the air disappears abruptly, and Cornelia's voice begins to sound booming and indecipherable, as if in a stone cave. It's bad when there aren't any windows. Or maybe it doesn't have anything to do with windows. I suddenly feel as if a tiny portal into a long-forgotten abyss is opening slightly. And from there, from the abyss, a draft of panic is reaching out in place of the air. In this room, with this woman—there's nothing to breathe.

This woman is the angel of death.

This room is a burial vault.

In this room, I looked into the basket with a cold, hurt baby. In this room... No, not in this one. I shake off the hallucination. This room simply looks like that other one. But it's not that one. Not that one... The portal slams shut. And once more I hear what Cornelia is saying to me.

> ... I call them by name if the parents have a name for them. Or else, sometimes there are nicknames, like Little Star. Sometimes the women, having heard what I do, also say something to them. And these are good moments, later they'll remember them all their lives. Life, of course, goes on... Usually, several hours are enough for a woman to be with her dead baby and "release" him. But a few come back again later. For that reason, we have a special refrigerator with a fan and temperature sensor. The babies are kept naked there to prevent mold. If the mother wants to see her baby, it's the midwife's task—at any hour of the day—to dress the baby and show him to the mother...

... A little later, after the interview is over, Cornelia will lead me through the maternity department and show me, among other objects of note, that same refrigerator. It's small. Entirely ordinary to look at. With a temperature sensor showing plus-four degrees Celsius. She will ingenuously throw open the door in front of me and suggest that I look inside. There, inside, I'll see two white plates, and on the plates will be two wrapped bundles that look like pieces of cheese packed in paper. But I'll know that this isn't cheese, and the air will disappear again for a while. "Here, the temperature is always between three and five degrees," Cornelia will say, with pride. "We take them out of here, dress them, and show them to the woman, if she wants to see her baby." They take them out of here. Out of an ordinary refrigerator.

They took mine out of the same kind of refrigerator, once. And dressed him. And laid him in a basket. And showed him to me.

... And a few want to see their children years later—in that case, we have a photo and footprints. We always try to take a photo and footprints and give them to the parents at discharge. We give them to them in a sealed envelope—just in case they don't want to see the photo, but so that they'll have the chance to pull out the photo and look at it any time.

Do you believe in God?

Yes, I do. Some women don't believe, but all the same, they want to baptize their children or bless them, if they're born dead. They feel easier after that. At the hospital, we have members of the clergy, but if for some reason a member of the clergy isn't available, and the matter is urgent, I may baptize a child myself.

You?!

Yes. Midwives are permitted to baptize children. Or to conduct a blessing ceremony, if the child is born dead.

And is it possible to conduct that ceremony with a fetus? With a baby who's only twenty gestational weeks old?

Even at eleven weeks! You can conduct a ceremony with any baby. Fifteen years ago, it wasn't this way, but we secured this right for women and their babies. Because grief isn't any less just because the gestational age is lower.

And is there a "specialist" like you for stillborn babies at every maternity hospital in Germany?

No, but I'm working on it. For example, soon I'll conduct a four-week congress with the Protestant academy, and I've already found a home for it—a very bright place, with big windows... Midwives and medical personnel from all over Germany will come, and I'll conduct something like a course to improve their qualifications. I've already done one such set of seminars for colleagues on attending births with children who won't live. By the way, when we began exchanging experiences with midwives from East Germany, it turned out that, until the Berlin Wall fell, they simply threw such babies into a bucket of water. We here in West Germany were absolutely shocked at such a practice. We didn't do that even in the 1980s. In West Germany, we used this tactic: let the baby die on his own. But we usually carried him away from his mother into another room... And so, we were shocked by their tactics, and they were shocked by ours. We said to them that a bucket of water is very callous, and they said to us: "But the baby wasn't able to live!" Now, of course, none of that happens anywhere. But all the same, not everyone understands how to attend these births. And I have rich experience. So, I tell them how I help women psychologically, how I carry myself, what can be done, and what shouldn't be done. For example, it's a bad idea to use scented candles in the places where these births take place. For the rest of their lives, women will remember that scent and won't be able to bear it, it will be associated with the death of their child.

And how do you help women psychologically?

I try to do what I can for them. Some need me to hold their hand, or even hug them. At first, I thought that was too intimate, but if someone asks, that means it's really better. Therefore, I never refuse such requests. And on the contrary, I offer: "Do you want a hug?" Some want it, some don't, and some women are in doubt and say: "I don't know." I answer: "Shall we try it?" And I hug her. Especially if she doesn't have a partner, or the partner is in bad shape, if he's frozen... It's also good to help massage a woman's feet. Even just laying your hands on the feet and keeping them there for ten to fifteen minutes, that helps a lot! For a few, an embrace is too much, but touching the feet is just right. For a few, tactile contact, on the contrary, is unacceptable—I take that calmly. I'm no one to them—not anyone dear, not a friend. I'm a stranger. But sometimes, it's precisely a stranger who can help in such a situation... I also often give the women whose births I attend some kind of small item, a little knickknack so they can tug at it, squeeze it, sometimes it's very important for them to hold something in their hand. And later, they lay that thing in the baby's grave—or keep it their whole lives as a memento.

What might that item be?

Well, for example, these colored pebbles. And this pendant—hang it in the window, and when the sun catches it, a hundred little rainbows appear in the room. Strangely enough, these small items can do a great deal, they can help a lot. But if a woman doesn't want them, if it seems to her that these are just stupid objects, I don't force the issue, I take the things away. Would you like these? I brought them especially for you.

... She holds out a pendant and two pebbles, a deep blue one and a red one, much like those that the child psychologist gave my Little Badger: "... this will be your strength, and this, your happiness...." And I take my strength, my happiness, and a hundred rainbows from the hands of the woman who works as the angel of death. From hands that didn't embrace me, but have embraced so many others like me.

Appendix
Statistics for Pregnancy Termination in Germany and Russia

Shortly after our interview, Dr. Christine Klapp sent me the link to publicly available statistics on abortion in Germany, including the termination of pregnancy for medical reasons. I wasn't able to find similarly detailed statistics for Russia (there are publicly available data from the Russian Federal State Statistics Service, Rosstat, on abortion by region and age of the woman, but no information about reasons for termination or length of pregnancy; I wasn't able to obtain the necessary statistics from doctors because of the inaccessibility of those doctors). Nevertheless, the German statistics may be useful for Russia, too. For example, insofar as climate and ecological conditions in Russia and Germany are to a certain degree similar, and the populations don't differ too much genetically or phenotypically, in these two countries we can expect approximately the same percentage of intrauterine mutations. Therefore, I suppose that German statistics concerning termination for medical reasons might, by and large, also be applied to Russian reality, adjusted for population size. The population in Germany is on the order of 81.3 million people, and in Russia is 146.5 million, that is, almost two times larger.

However, with regard to the total number of abortions, most of which are abortions at up to twelve weeks "in lieu of contraception," the correlation of percentages between Germany and Russia suggested above doesn't work. According to the statistics of Rosstat (see below), the total number of abortions in the Russian Federation in 2014 exceeded the total number of abortions in Germany by almost ten times.

Statistics for Medical Abortions in Germany[1]

All pregnancy terminations	2013	2014	2015
	102,802	99,715	99,237
Grounds for termination			
On medical grounds	3,703	3,594	3,879
As the result of a crime (rape)	20	41	20
Ordinary abortion (as a means of contraception)	99,079	96,080	95,338
Length of pregnancy at time of termination			
Up to 12 weeks	100,002	96,935	96,442
From 12 to 21 weeks	2,238	2,196	2,161
22 weeks and greater	562	584	634
Living children before abortion			
No children before abortion	40,506	39,261	38,793
One child before abortion	26,718	25,316	24,869
Two children before abortion	23,711	23,159	23,111
Three children before abortion	8,260	8,310	8,533
Four children before abortion	2,431	2,509	2,597
Five or more children before abortion	1,176	1,160	1,334

[1] Data from the site of the Federal Statistical Office of Germany: https://www.destatis.de/DEZahlenFaktenGesellschaftStaat/Gesundheit/Schwangerschaftsabbrueche Tabellen Rechtliche Begruendung.html [NOTE: The link in the original text appears to be incorrect. An updated version of this material can be found at https://www.destatis.de/EN/Themes/Society-Environment/Health/Abortions/Tables/legal-statement.html—*trans.*]

Statistics for Pregnancy Termination in Russia for 2014[2]

All pregnancy terminations in the Russian Federation: 929,963
This sum includes:

Age	Number of pregnancy terminations
Up to age 14	354
Ages 15–17	9,902
Ages 18–19	28,715
Ages 20–24	173,390
Ages 25–29	263,282
Ages 30–34	232,717
Ages 35–39	157,918
Ages 40–44	58,927
Ages 45–49	4,607
Age 50 and older	151

[2] Data from the site of the Russian Federal State Statistics Service (Rosstat): http://www.gks.ru/. [NOTE: The citation is incomplete in the original. This table can be accessed as a downloadable .doc file at https://www.gks.ru/bgd/regl/b15_34/Main.htm (> Состояние здоровья населения > Состояние здоровья женщин > Прерывание беременности (аборты) по возрастным группам)—*trans.*]

About the Author

Anna Starobinets was born in 1978 in Moscow, Russia. She is a journalist and contributor to a number of publications, including *Expert* and *Russian Reporter*, writing on cultural issues. She is also a successful scriptwriter; several of her scripts have been turned into feature films and TV shows. *The Awkward Age*, her debut collection of short stories, has been translated into a number of languages, including English (Hesperus). Her prose works include the novel *Refuge F/A* (2007); a collection of short novels, *Cold Spell* (2008); a tie-in, *The First Squad: The Moment of Truth* (2010); a collection of short stories, *Icarus Gland* (2013); and a number of books for children, including the internationally bestselling series Beastly Crimes Books, now being adapted into an animation series. All of her novels have been nominated for the National Bestseller Prize in Russia. In 2014 Starobinets won the National Bestseller Prize in the Young Writers category; she was awarded the Eurocon Prize in 2018. For more on Starobinets, please visit her Web page at https://starobinets.ru/eng/.

About the Translator

Katherine E. Young is the author of *Day of the Border Guards*, 2014 Miller Williams Arkansas Poetry Prize finalist, and *Woman Drinking Absinthe* (forthcoming 2021). Her translations of Russian-language poetry and prose include *Farewell, Aylis* by Azerbaijani political prisoner Akram Aylisli and *Blue Birds and Red Horses* and *Two Poems* by Inna Kabysh. Young is a 2020 Arlington, VA, individual artist grantee and a 2017 National Endowment for the Arts translation fellow. From 2016-2018 she served as the inaugural poet laureate for Arlington, VA. For further information, please go to https://katherine-young-poet.com.